STAY OFF
MY OPERATING TABLE

A Heart Surgeon's
Metabolic Health Guide
to Lose Weight, Prevent
Disease, and Feel Your
Best Every Day

PRAISE FOR *STAY OFF MY OPERATING TABLE*

Stay Off My Operating Table is a must-read. This is the book for any physician or patient who wants to prevent disease if possible and to otherwise improve outcomes. Dr. Ovadia understands the central role metabolic health plays in the body, knowledge which enables him to keep potential future cardiac patients off his operating table. I am sharing this book with other doctors at the USC Keck School of Medicine so they can learn how diet affects everything we do in medicine.

ROBERT LUFKIN, MD
Chief of Head Neck Imaging/Neuroradiology, Prohealth Advanced Imaging Network
& Clinical Professor of Radiology, USC Keck School of Medicine

Working in clinical medicine for more than twenty years has demonstrated to me that we often overlook the root cause of chronic disease in an effort to manage symptoms. I firmly believe that if we could help identify the real etiologies and reasons for chronic illness, and the lifestyle contributors to inflammation, insulin resistance, etc., we would have a much healthier population. Dr. Philip Ovadia's book brilliantly identifies how best to empower our current medical establishment to help reverse current statistics and metabolic inflexibility.

CYNTHIA THURLOW
Nurse Practitioner, Intermittent Fasting and Nutrition Expert, and Two-Time TEDx Speaker

Like Dr. Philip Ovadia, I struggled with obesity throughout my life. I, too, learned almost too late that the root of many chronic diseases is not too high a fat or protein intake but often too many carbohydrates. Today, both Dr. Ovadia and I recommend patients and clients focus on getting meals that are rich in protein and healthy fats. For a system that makes metabolically balanced nutrition easy and sustainable, get *Stay Off My Operating Table*.

DR. TRO KALAYJIAN
Internal Medicine & Obesity Medicine Physician

Most so-called "health experts" have no idea what they're talking about. In fact, their advice usually results in you getting sicker, fatter, and angrier. And you're left with no clue about what to do different. Dr. Philip Ovadia changes everything. Not only is he an actual doctor who understands the problems with our sick-care system, he knows how the human body actually works. In *Stay Off My Operating Table*, Dr. Ovadia shows you how to get your metabolic health right and, in turn, get everything else right. Your weight, your blood sugar, your blood pressure, your cholesterol and triglycerides, your energy, everything. I recommend this book to anyone who is sick of being lied to by self-styled fitness gurus and professional dieticians who don't know the first thing about being fit or healthy.

VINNIE TORTORICH
Author, *Fitness Confidential*

This is a comprehensive book on metabolic health—a book that covers all aspects of good health and addresses common myths which have contributed to ill health not only in the United States but also globally. The often-complicated science is explained in an accessible language that would appeal to all. It's the perfect book to gift to a hesitant friend or a confused family member. My extended family members are going to receive a copy each!

NAYIRI MISSISSIAN
Managing Director, ntsprofessionaltranslations.com
Nutrition Researcher & Coach, lowcarbandfasting.com

If only I had read this as a young doctor! Instead, I wasted years using lifelong medication instead of lifestyle medicine, particularly a real food, low-carb diet as advocated in these pages. I spent years blindly following the myths debunked in this book. Since "seeing the light" I have helped over one hundred patients achieve drug free Type 2 diabetes remission. Don't wait, read it now!

DR. DAVID UNWIN, FRCGP, RCGP
National Champion for Collaborative Care and Support Planning in Obesity & Diabetes,
2016 NHS Innovator of the Year

Dr. Ovadia's brave message is one that needs to be shouted from ORs everywhere: Many surgeries are completely preventable, and in order to stay off the operating table, we need to take responsibility for our own health, diets, and lifestyle by proactively addressing the root causes of disease. Spoiler alert: It all starts with eating real, whole food. Dr. Ovadia gives us the framework for how to improve our metabolic health, with flexible plans for different dietary preferences. This book will leave you empowered to take your metabolic health into your own hands so you can live your most vibrant, empowered, and healthy life.

CASEY MEANS, MD
Co-Founder and Chief Medical Officer of Levels

In a time where our world grapples with a health matter where morbidity relates to metabolic syndrome and insulin resistance, it is clear we as a people have both ignored warnings for decades and are in need of true and honest leadership from the medical profession. With the release of *Stay Off My Operating Table*, Dr. Ovadia has supplied our world a tour-de-force blueprint for both the average citizen and the medical professional to understand the role of metabolic syndrome and how to right the storm and nurture a legacy of health in their family as well as across the globe. Thank you, Dr. Ovadia. I strongly encourage all to read *Stay Off My Operating Table*.

JOHN K. DAVIES
JKD Asset Management

STAY OFF
MY OPERATING TABLE

A Heart Surgeon's
Metabolic Health Guide
to Lose Weight, Prevent
Disease, and Feel Your
Best Every Day

PHILIP OVADIA MD

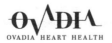

OVADIA HEART HEALTH

Cover and content design by Houseal Creative

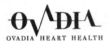

Ovadia Heart Health LLC
204 37th Ave #289
St Petersburg FL 33704
ovadiahearthealth.com
Send feedback to **philip.ovadia@ovadiahearthealth.com**

Publisher's Cataloging-In-Publication Data

Names: Ovadia, Philip, author.
Title: Stay off my operating table : a heart surgeon's metabolic health guide to lose weight, prevent disease, and feel your best every day / Philip Ovadia.
Description: St. Petersburg, FL : Ovadia Heart Health LLC, [2021] | Includes bibliographical references.
Identifiers: ISBN 9781737818205 (hardcover) | ISBN 9781737818212 (softcover) | ISBN 9781737818229 (ebook)
Subjects: LCSH: Medicine, Preventive. | Metabolism--Disorders--Prevention. | Weight loss. | Diet therapy. | Metabolic manifestations of general diseases.
Classification: LCC RA425 .O93 2021 (print) | LCC RA425 (ebook) | DDC 613--dc23

Special discounts for bulk sales are available.
Please contact **philip.ovadia@ovadiahearthealth.com**

To my amazing wife, Shelly, whose support and inspiration has allowed me to aim for the stars, and to my daughters, Eva and Layla, who provide the "why" for me to give them a better world.

TELL ME WHAT YOU THINK

Let other readers know what you
thought of *Stay Off My Operating Table*.
Please write an honest review for this book
at your favorite online bookshop.

CONTENTS

PART II
PRINCIPLES OF METABOLIC HEALTH

PART III
HOW TO EAT METABOLICALLY HEALTHY

METABOLIC HEALTH TRACKING SYSTEM

This action-oriented course is a **companion** to Dr. Ovadia's *Stay Off My Operating Table*. The activities, spreadsheets, trackers, shopping lists, food guides, and downloads in this course help you quickly, correctly, easily, and sustainably follow Dr. Ovadia's metabolic health advice so you can:

- Track your 5 metabolic health markers and make continual progress
- **Put the 7 metabolic health principles into practice every day**
- Turn metabolically healthy eating into a habit
- **Find the exact foods at the grocery fast**
- Read and follow legitimate medical experts to support your journey
- **Remember which metabolically unhealthy foods to sub out of your diet**
- Know how to talk to any doctor about metabolic health

Make your health goals happen with the **Metabolic Health Tracking System**. The course retails for $99, but you get **50% off** when you use discount code **COURSE**.

ovadiahearthealth.com/course

SAVE
50%

ENTER CODE: **COURSE**

FOREWORD

by JACK MURPHY

I met Dr. Philip Ovadia when he joined the Liminal Order, my all-men's professional network. He came with a big idea—starting a telehealth practice to help people become metabolically healthier. In his practice as a heart surgeon, he saw firsthand the dangers of unhealthy lifestyles, particularly food choices. Dr. Ovadia told me he wanted to keep people out of his operating room by giving them the resources they need to be healthy now, instead of after undergoing surgery.

That's how I knew Dr. Ovadia was the real deal. What kind of surgeon wants to limit his customers? Honest ones, that's who. The good kind. I had recently had negative experiences with orthopedic surgeons who had all wanted to put me under the knife right away. In reality, physical therapy was the answer. So when I heard Dr. Ovadia was a man of health and integrity, I immediately wanted to support him. Today, many Liminal Order members are Dr. Ovadia's private clients, myself included. I recommend his telehealth services without reservation. But if you'd like a preview of what the good doctor is all about, read *Stay Off My Operating Table*.

This book gives you the knowledge and tools to become healthier, happier, and even wealthier. People who are metabolically healthy feel great, look great, live longer, and have more productive lives than those who don't. Metabolic health puts you in a special category of people who take control and elevate yourself to a new level. Dr. Ovadia's advice can take inches off your waist and put years on your life. Who doesn't want that? I know I do.

Dr. Ovadia is no longer a new acquaintance with big ideas. He's now a trusted friend, my personal physician, and an author with a powerful message. Stay off this man's operating table. Read this book, heed the words, and join us in an active rewarding life filled with many years and even more memories.

— Jack Murphy

PART I

THE STATE OF
METABOLIC HEALTH

STAY OFF MY OPERATING TABLE

I couldn't save her.

She should not have needed to be saved.

Two months before I began writing this book, I got called into the hospital for a surgical emergency. Corinne, a thirty-nine-year-old mother, arrived at the ER minutes earlier, presenting symptoms of an aortic aneurysm and dissection. That's when the blood vessel leading out of the heart tears. The torn wall of the blood vessel fills with blood intended for the organs, the limbs, and the brain. Abnormal blood flow like this carries a 30 percent mortality rate before the patient even reaches the hospital.

We had no time to waste. Corinne's only hope was rescue via the operating room, but the outcome looked grim as I spoke with her family. Corinne was still conscious as we wheeled her back for surgery.

"Will I be OK?" she asked me, fists clenched white at her sides.

TV doctors and the screenwriters behind them always know the perfect one-liner to deliver in a rush. Out here in the real world, when someone asks you—a member of the most trusted profession in the world—whether they will survive their medical emergency, no one perfect answer emerges. So you tell the truth. That and my two decades of cardiac surgery experience are all I could offer this woman.

"The damage could be severe, but we won't know until we go in," I said as calmly as I could. "If it is severe, there could also be damage elsewhere."

"Can you fix what's wrong?"

I took a breath and gave my honest assessment.

"I'll do everything I can."

"OK."

That was Corinne's last word to me. From the start of the surgery, I could see the damage was catastrophic. The tear in her blood vessel was so extensive, no routine repair would work. We knew that the longer we operated, more damage was being done. During parts of the operation, we temporarily interrupt blood flow to the brain and the body. The patient is essentially dead at that point, and we hope that we can bring them back to life.

That's not the harshest truth about the procedure. By the time a patient makes it to emergency surgery for an aortic aneurysm and dissection, it's sometimes too late. Delayed surgery isn't to blame, the tear itself is. Imagine a sailboat headed toward a raging thunderstorm on the horizon. The ship's only hope is its ability to steer away from a sailor's worst nightmare. Now imagine the sail is torn and the rudder broken. Onward the ship bobs in the waves into darkness. Even the world's most skilled navigators shudder at the thought.

That's how I felt with Corinne's life in my hands. For ten straight hours, from nightfall through morning rush hour, my team and I tried every tactic we knew. The mortality rate for aortic dissection surgery is as high as 20 percent, a statistic I failed to keep out of my mind. Of course, without surgery, nearly 100 percent of patients die. Compare these numbers to a more routine open-heart surgery, coronary artery bypass surgery, which carries a 2 percent mortality rate.

The truth had sunk in by dawn. Corinne had already been dying when she walked into the ER. She seemed alert during our conversation, but her body had already been shutting down on her. Still, my team and I fought like mad to give Corinne's heart every last chance medical science had to offer. In the end, no repair held. The high blood pressure and obesity I saw in Corinne's medical history had, years earlier, set her on a course we could not change.

I remember cleaning up after those ten gloomy hours. Minutes before I'd deliver the world's worst news to Corinne's children, husband, and parents, I stood alone in the washroom. I scrubbed my hands. And kept scrubbing. Kept washing, kept rinsing, kept soaping up. Over and over and over. The tactful, compassionate speech I'd give her family wrote itself in my head. So did a tweet. That would have to wait.

Walking toward the waiting area, seeing Corinne's kids shoot to their feet at the sight of me, I swallowed hard. The one message I most wanted to share with Corinne's family was the only one I knew wouldn't help:
It didn't have to be this way.

I offered the most sympathy I could. I'll spare the details and just say this—it was the toughest conversation I'd ever had. How do you explain to a child why her young mother left with you, the doctor, but didn't come back?

I stayed with Corinne's family longer than I usually do. Soon it seemed obvious my presence was no longer helpful. So I quietly exited to look for an empty utility closet. I just needed to think. Process. I also needed to get this all off my chest. So I sent this update to my online following of cardiologists, general practitioners, and healthcare professionals.

> Difficult night into morning. Nearly 10 hours of surgery and was unable to save a woman in her 30s who presented after years of untreated hypertension/poor metabolic health with an aortic aneurysm and dissection. Healthcare needs to do better at promoting metabolic health!

I may be a doctor whose specialty is the heart, but I see the whole person. More than anything, what we put in our bodies determines when life itself leaves them. The tear in Corinne's blood vessel was the last in a long series of medical failures that compounded to create a fatal and irreversible problem. Corinne could have saved herself if she'd known how, but the system failed her. She'd been morbidly obese for years, according to her chart. Her doctors had thrown a range of medications at her to manage the high blood pressure. And she'd taken them all. But the doctors and the drugs never addressed the underlying causes. No one had blunt conversations with Corinne about how to take care of herself, how and what to eat so she'd lower her blood pressure, lose the weight, and stay off the surgical table. There were so many opportunities to prevent death at age thirty-nine. At least . . . there should have been.

The real life-saving surgery would have been Corinne's own intervention ten years earlier, not a couple of hours after she began having trouble breathing. If Corinne had learned about metabolic health, what was happening inside her body, and how obesity and hypertension can permanently tear the heart, she might have been able to live past eighty. Her children might not have lost their mother so early in life. At the time of their mother's passing, two of them were under the age of four.

Corinne and people like her simply follow their doctors' advice. But it doesn't keep them from the operating table. Corinne had high blood pressure. She was overweight and had diabetes. Yet she was on all the medications and took them faithfully after they were prescribed. Still, she passed away. Heart disease is the leading cause of death in the United States. But the medical establishment just shrugs and says, "These things happen. Next patient."

After speaking with Corinne's family, I drove home bitterly angry. Not at her, no. Not at all. She'd merely done what the system told her to do. She'd followed orders. I was livid because her death was 100 percent preventable. For the first time in my surgical career, I made the heart-metabolism connection. And in an unforgettable way.

Aortic dissections are not necessary, I remember thinking that morning. I had access to information few doctors do because I had been on a health journey of my own.

I'm a surgeon. But I'll be the first to tell you—to beg you—to do whatever it takes to never, ever need me. Please stay off my operating table. Through this book, I hope to write myself out of a career. I want to make lifesaving heart surgeries unnecessary and untimely demises obsolete.

I don't want to see even one more preventable death because the situation held off until it was too late to be saved.

This book isn't just about heart health. It's about the whole body and all the diseases that we just take for granted. Someone dies of diabetes, of stroke, of Alzheimer's, and we shrug and say, "Aww, too bad. But hey, it happens." But *why*? *Why* does it happen?

Only **metabolic health** has the answer—and the prevention. The brutal truth is, our medical care system is not built to broadcast that answer, much less comprehend it. The system addresses only the symptoms of metabolic health problems as they arise, rarely if ever resolving the underlying causes.

As you're reading this book, maybe you've been diagnosed with type 2 diabetes or an autoimmune condition. There are signs of inflammation. Your joints hurt due to obesity, and you're unable to play with your grandkids. It could be that you're a survivor of heart failure and are looking for answers on what to do next. Or you're a young person who's struggled with weight and wants to learn how to avoid medical issues later on.

I want you to know I've been on both sides of the office visit, both as a heart surgeon and as a patient. I know what it's like to struggle and wonder if I would one day end up on the operating table.

HOW I LOST 100 POUNDS (AND FORGOT EVERYTHING I LEARNED ABOUT FAT)

I had never heard about the wider world of metabolic health before Gary Taubes gave a speech at a medical conference. The talk was based on his new book at that time, *The Case Against Sugar*. Taubes lectured not just about obesity, which we all knew was a problem, but also about the causes of it. I'd never heard that there could be a deeper issue than the common-sense "too many calories in, too few calories out" weight gain equation. Hearing Taubes speak about the addictive dangers of sugar, I realized I'd never been given the full picture of how fat works—and why it's so hard for cardiac patients to get their health back.

After the conference, I devoured Taubes's books. I was hungry for more. I needed to learn everything I could about this new, unfamiliar topic—metabolic health. I read low-carb books and keto diet books and everything else I could find with "metabolic" anything in the table of contents. Over time, a new way to help patients emerged, an education program that could teach the patients coming into my clinic how to save themselves before they even needed surgery. My nutrition and wellness coaching practice was born.

Let's stop and define exactly what I mean by metabolic health—it's how your body uses the food you put into it. It affects everything. If the body is not running on the proper fuels, and if there is an excess of toxic substances, that damages all the organs.[1] The fact we've become obese is a reflection of other processes that accompany poor metabolic health: inflammation that damages blood vessels, insulin resistance building to the point of needing medication, and so on.[2,3,4,5] In fact, we often identify poor metabolic health with insulin resistance, because that's the easiest measurement of it in your body. But obesity, inflammation, and high blood pressure are all indicators as well, along with a host of unseen damage taking place below the surface that doesn't become visible until people are on my table and it's too late.

Insulin resistance has been known and described since the 1960s. That's approximately sixty years, but our treatments still focus on handling the outcomes from long-term resistance instead of addressing the root causes and preventing the damage in the first place.

---

1   Romilly E. Hodges and Deanna M. Minich, "Modulation of Metabolic Detoxification Pathways Using Foods and Food-Derived Components: A Scientific Review with Clinical Application," *Journal of Nutrition and Metabolism*, (2015), https://doi.org/10.1155/2015/760689.

2   Atilla Engin, "The Definition and Prevalence of Obesity and Metabolic Syndrome," in *Obesity and Lipotoxicity*, ed. Ayse Basak Engin and Atilla Engin (Springer, 2017), 1-17.

3   K. Esposito and D. Giugliano, "The Metabolic Syndrome and Inflammation: Association or Causation?" *Nutrition, Metabolism & Cardiovascular Diseases* 14, no. 5 (2004): 228-232, https://doi.org/10.1016/S0939-4753(04)80048-6.

4   Johnathan D. Tune, Adam G. Goodwill, Daniel J. Sassoon, and Kieren J. Mather, "Cardiovascular Consequences of Metabolic Syndrome," *Translational Research* 183 (2017): 57-70. https://doi.org/10.1016/j.trsl.2017.01.001.

5   "Metabolic Syndrome," Health, Johns Hopkins Medicine, accessed August 10, 2021, https://www.hopkinsmedicine.org/health/conditions-and-diseases/metabolic-syndrome.

People come to me with obesity, heart disease, diabetes, and other health conditions. What they—and even their doctors—don't understand is the root cause of metabolic health. Improve that, and everything else improves.

I know this from personal experience. I had been obese since childhood, and by the time I was forty, I was morbidly obese. That's right, I was one of those medical experts who was himself unhealthy. I had followed the advice, and it failed. In this case, it's because the metabolic health advice I had been taught—calories in, calories out—was basically useless. And I didn't yet understand the link between metabolic health and catastrophic outcomes.

Then I heard Gary Taubes's talk on sugar, and it all clicked for me. I cut sugars out of my diet, then carbs, then processed ingredients, then artificial ingredients, then vegetable and seed oils. I dropped one hundred pounds and reversed my prediabetic blood markers. I've maintained the weight loss using the tools I'll teach you in this book. But it all began with learning what I'd never been taught, even in medical school.

I no longer think, stress, or worry about food. When I was overweight I'd worry, "Is the cafeteria going to be open after this long surgery?" Now, if I'm hungry, I prepare my food simply, quickly, and cheaply. I don't spend a fortune on premium ingredients the way that people worry that "clean eating" is going to require. If I am hungry and food is not available, I've stored enough healthy nutrients in my body that I won't be starving. I can drive past all the fast-food temptations on my way home and eat a healthy meal I know will help me rather than threaten my life.

CARDIAC SURGEON, METABOLIC HEALTH ADVOCATE

Why on earth would I keep this knowledge to myself? Like I said, I'm a heart surgeon, but I'd rather put myself out of a job educating people than lose even one more patient who could have lived. So I've begun helping people ten years before they need surgery. With education, I can prevent them from ending up on my table, or being on insulin, or becoming obese, or any of the other catastrophic outcomes that our medical system just shrugs and accepts. My medical practice focused on metabolic health is my way of keeping people off my surgical table.

Here are just a few examples of changes I've helped coaching students make in their lives through metabolic health education.

One nurse anesthetist, fifty-two years old, lost fifty pounds in one year. He was able to put on his uniform from basic training when he was eighteen, and it fit for the first time since his twenties.

A couple who lost seventy combined pounds in just four months reported having more energy for their six kids. The wife talks about how much better she feels, even though she hasn't lost as much weight as she thought she would have to. The changes were noticeable even with small improvements.

I've worked with a host of men on testosterone replacement therapy. We wean them off their medications without them having low-T symptoms anymore, all because improving metabolic health improves testosterone levels.

Preventing heart disease is a ten- to twenty-year journey, but we've seen improved heart scans as people stop feeding themselves poison and give their body what it needs to thrive.

I've even helped people reverse type 2 diabetes, something the medical system will teach you is close to impossible.

Metabolic health has achieved medical miracles. What can it do for you?

THE LIFESAVING POWER OF METABOLIC HEALTH

I want to disseminate this information to as many people as possible. This is what medical professionals do with their own research. A book is a more effective way of disseminating this information to larger numbers of people, particularly the general public, who follow the dictates of trusted physicians. A book is also more concrete than a podcast or a talk I could give, though I've done plenty of both.

My objective is to provide the last diet book you'll ever need. This book presents a lifelong framework for healthy metabolic living. But I encourage you to listen to other advisors or read other books, and you may want to gather additional tips and advanced strategies. The reason people are dying young (or younger than they ought to) is that they just don't know what they're doing wrong. Arm yourself with knowledge, educate yourself about the problem, and live a longer, healthier life. I'm begging you: Do *not* stop educating yourself. Keep yourself off my operating table. Take back control of your health. Don't allow the medical system that no longer allows your doctor to take the time to talk with you to prevent you from being healthy.

The metabolic health plan I teach in this book is not your typical diet advice. That's by design, because we must get away from the typical advice that fails over and over. Instead, I'm going to teach you sustainable life changes to make that can save your life long term. There is no "Week One, Week Two" eating plan. There is no "thirty-day plan to track, then you're done." And I'm not going to give you checklists of specific foods to eat or to not eat. I'm going to give you a system anyone can use.

I see the anger, frustration, and hopelessness at the end of the line. I talk to patients post-op about their metabolic health and am greeted by skepticism, because these patients were already listening to doctors who gave them advice that resulted in them landing on my operating table. Their doctors failed them, probably because those doctors didn't even know the truth.

I wrote this book to make sure no one misses the truth ever again.

HOW TO USE THIS BOOK (LIKE YOU'VE NEVER USED ANOTHER DIET BOOK)

The metabolic health principles in this book work when nothing else has. I know, because I tried everything else myself when I was struggling to lose weight. This is the system that finally helped me get fit, get healthy, and erased my growing medical problems. It's easier to follow and less restrictive than anything else I tried, and it doesn't involve a list of must-buys marketed by the diet designer.

The truth is, if all those other diet plans actually worked, they'd go out of business. All their shakes and supplements and thirty-day programs would cure obesity, and every person would be too healthy to need those products ever again. But obesity is worse than ever before. I tell clients and patients improving their metabolic health that they can also expect to:

- Lose weight
- Get energy
- Find mental clarity
- Stop feeling bloated
- No longer need certain medications
- Become decisive
- Look good and feel great
- Enjoy their clothes again
- Improve their interpersonal relationships, become more themselves, and be more present
- Suffer fewer hormonal swings than before and enjoy a more stable mood
- Face no more fighting with their spouse and family about dieting

Consider the subtle benefits of improved metabolic health. When you lose weight, you become more confident. Becoming metabolically healthy has given me the confidence to author this book and start my own private consulting practice, all without being tired.

It feels like a miracle to finally get unstuck. You can get more respect and stop slinking away and withdrawing because you have to admit another diet failure to your family and friends when they see you gained back all that weight you lost. Ending that cycle of shame is almost as big a relief as taking the stress off your joints.

Do you feel tired all the time? When you control your metabolic health, you can maintain predictable, sustained levels of energy throughout the day, with no crashing. When I was overweight, I'd get exhausted just from work and routinely fell asleep at three in the afternoon for a nap. Now I can work in the operating room from eight o'clock in the morning to eight o'clock at night, spend a couple of hours on a live webinar, and work on my business, all without feeling exhausted.

You can achieve all of these effects in your own life. You just need to follow the system I'll present in the chapters ahead.

BUT FIRST, WE'VE GOT SOME DEBUNKING TO DO

To achieve the full metabolic health overhaul, we need to first unlearn the "facts" about nutrition, fitness, dieting, and the medical system that pushes them. Understanding what is false takes you more than halfway to the truth.

People like Corinne meet the fate they do in part because of the myths we're about to debunk. It's no direct fault of their own. Even family and friends cosign untrue, unhelpful beliefs that ultimately result in long-term medications, expensive surgeries, and golden years consumed by poor health.

The pervading narrative is so strong that you need a counter-narrative. That's up next.

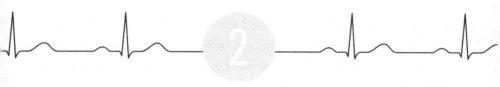

THE TWELVE MYTHS THEY
WANT US TO BELIEVE

For as long as I can remember, I was overweight. As a child, as a teenager, as a student at medical school, and even as a cardiac surgeon.

This was despite growing up in a household that followed official government health guidelines. I was an active child who played sports. My parents bought margarine, diet soda, and low-fat milk. We ate grains at every meal, beginning with cereal for breakfast. We followed the guidelines of the USDA and the food pyramid.

Yet I was always overweight. And I got heavier as I progressed through college and medical school.

While making rounds at the hospital at the age of twenty-seven, I was convinced that I was suffering a heart attack. I wasn't—it was probably just severe heartburn—but it scared me into action anyway. It was time to lose weight.

For months, I tracked everything I ate. I followed the "calories in, calories out" principle that I learned at school, making sure I was consuming less than I was burning. I also exercised for many hours each day. And it worked: I lost fifty pounds!

Of course, that's not the end of the story. You wouldn't be reading this if it was. Like many other people, I put all of that weight back on, and then added some more. Both of my parents were obese and underwent gastric bypass surgery, so I resigned myself to being genetically destined for obesity. This was another concept taught to me at medical school.

Obesity stared me in the face every day, both in the mirror and in the hospital. I treated obese and diabetic people on a daily basis, and each time I gave them the same advice that I'd always been told: "Eat less. Move more. Choose low-fat foods." I believed this was the correct advice, and I continued to follow it myself. Over the years I tried everything, including Weight Watchers and Nutrisystem. Sure, I always lost weight, but I always put it back on. Plus extra.

Then, in 2015, things really changed for me—and I owe it all to my wife. She had suffered from severe heartburn since giving birth to our daughters, and she decided to try avoiding gluten to see if it helped. I joined her in a bid to be supportive, and I was stunned to discover that I immediately felt better. I had more energy, and some of my excess weight disappeared.

Sometimes life presents strange coincidences, and I experienced one a short while later. At a medical conference, I listened to low-carbohydrate diet advocate Gary Taubes deliver an alternative explanation for the underlying cause of obesity: sugar specifically and carbohydrates generally. His talk led me to his books, which inspired me to cut my own carbohydrate intake. This one decision changed my life.

Do you spend all day thinking about food? Feeling hungry from the moment you wake up until you go to bed? I did. But not anymore. For the first time since I could remember, I did not think about food constantly. I lost those one hundred pounds, and I *finally* kept them off.

Today, I'm in the best shape of my life. Physically, I have never been fitter or felt better, and I have a mental clarity that I have never experienced before. Some say that life begins at forty, and that was absolutely true in my case. My entire life had been spent battling my weight; focusing on it, losing it, and gaining it. Then, with a simple decision to support my wife and read a few books, that battle ended with victory.

As you might expect, this led me on a quest. I had serious questions:

- How did this happen?
- Why is this not in the food pyramid?
- Why was this not taught to me in medical school?

I researched obsessively into the effects of food on health. I learned that much of what I had been taught at school was based on a number of fallacies. And I came to realize that our poor diets cause poor metabolic health, which is why we suffer from so many chronic diseases.

Processed food is intentionally engineered to encourage people to eat more, creating a vicious cycle. Worse, our healthcare environment is overly focused on prescribing medicines and treating the symptoms of a condition instead of addressing the root cause and preventing the issue in the first place.

It became my mission to help people who were fighting the same battle that I had won. That's what put me on the path to writing this book.

EVEN DOCTORS BELIEVE THESE MYTHS!

I had a lot to unlearn about what it means to be healthy. If I as a physician had a lot to unlearn, you can bet the general public does, too.

For example, I was led to believe that margarine is "heart healthy." It's not. It's poison. Because of its artificially produced fat profile, our body is not able to consume its nutritional value.[6,7] The highly processed fat in margarine disrupts the mitochondria. Mitochondria are the powerhouses of the cell. They're the basic machinery that your body runs on, and if it doesn't run correctly, your body suffers.[8] You notice the effects in your

---

6   "Butter vs. Margarine," Harvard Health Publishing, Harvard Medical School, last updated January 29, 2020, https://www.health.harvard.edu/staying-healthy/butter-vs-margarine.
7   Scott Cuthbert, "Ask Dr Scott: I Can't Believe I'm Using Margarine," Pulp, last updated October 12, 2017, https://pueblopulp.com/i-cant-believe-im-using-margarine-ask-dr-scott/.
8   Huei-Fen Jheng, Pei-Jane Tsai, Syue-Maio Guo, Li-Hua Kuo, Cherng-Shyang Chang, Ih-Jen Su, Chuang-Rung Chang, Yau-Sheng Tsai, "Mitochondrial Fission Contributes to Mitochondrial Dysfunction and Insulin Resistance in Skeletal Muscle," *Molecular and Cellular Biology* 32, no. 2 (2020). https://doi.org/10.1128/MCB.05603-11.

metabolism first, when your body starts storing more fat than it should. Soon other chronic medical problems arise, like diabetes and heart disease.[9]

The "margarine is heart healthy" myth is just one of many you have to unlearn if you're going to get (and stay) healthy. But don't beat yourself up for believing these myths. As a highly educated adult, I believed all of them. So did my parents. They did everything they believed was right and still raised an unhealthy child who went on to become an unhealthy heart surgeon. There's no shame in believing what we were all taught. Now that I've learned the truth, I'm going to help you learn it, too.

Let's start the unlearning right now by shattering the twelve deadliest food lies you've been taught.

MYTH #1: "ONLY OBESE PEOPLE ARE METABOLICALLY UNHEALTHY."

To address this myth, we need to define "metabolic health."

Good metabolic health means your metabolism is correctly utilizing the energy you give it, mostly via food. When our metabolism functions optimally, we eat a certain amount of food and use that to build and repair our tissues, power our daily activities, and store a little in case food isn't available later. Our ancestors often had times when food was unavailable; hence the need for a storage mechanism. Our bodies have actually evolved to endure periods of food unavailability. But we no longer tap into those energy stores, so they accumulate excessively. *That* is poor metabolic health.

Yes, obesity is one obvious indicator of poor metabolic health, but using weight as the sole marker is not only unhelpful, it's dangerous. Some people are what is often referred to as "skinny fat" or TOFI (thin outside, fat inside) by medical professionals. TOFI individuals suffer from many

---

9   "Metabolic Syndrome," Patient Care & Health Information, Mayo Clinic, last accessed August 10, 2021, https://www.mayoclinic.org/diseases-conditions/metabolic-syndrome/symptoms-causes/syc-20351916#:~:text=Metabolic%20syndrome%20is%20a%20cluster,abnormal%20cholesterol%20or%20 triglyceride%20levels.

of the same health issues as a person who struggles with obesity. They also have poor metabolic health, it's just not as obvious.[10]

Everyone has a different personal fat threshold, which is how overweight they can get before their metabolic health goes off the rails. Sometimes that turns them obese, and other times it destroys their internal health without any external signs. That's why using external obesity is not a useful indicator of metabolic health. In science, we even have a term for this—metabolically healthy obesity.[11]

We haven't always understood the deeper issues with metabolic health. Fifty years ago, the experts assumed that poor metabolic health was the result of carrying excess fat. To prevent excess fat, eat fewer fats, right? This led to the myth that you're automatically healthy if you don't have excess fat. Now that we understand a person can look skinny but still develop diabetes, it's time to let go of the tired stereotype that only obese people are unhealthy.

MYTH #2: "THE FOOD PYRAMID IS GOOD FOR YOU."

The food pyramid was designed around fifty years ago under the same initiative that equated poor metabolic health with obesity. The creators targeted the heart disease epidemic by limiting the amount of fat a person should eat. The stated goal of the food pyramid is to keep people healthy, specifically by preventing them from becoming obese. But as you just learned, preventing obesity doesn't keep people healthy. In fact, it's the other way around: maintaining good metabolic health prevents health issues, including obesity. As I learned from my own experience and the experiences of the patients I've treated, the high-carbohydrate, low-fat

---

10 Norbert Stefan, "Metabolically Healthy and Unhealthy Normal Weight and Obesity," *Endocrinology and Metabolism* 35, no. 3 (2020): 487-493. https://doi.org/10.3803/EnM.2020.301.
11 Jennifer Couzin-Franke, "Obesity Doesn't Always Mean Ill Health. Here's What Scientists Are Learning," *Science*, July 29, 2021, https://www.sciencemag.org/news/2021/07/obesity-doesn-t-always-mean-ill-health-here-s-what-scientists-are-learning.

diet that the food pyramid recommends keeps people in poor metabolic health.[12,13]

We've had the same food pyramid for fifty years. Just look how the American diet has shifted. We eat more carbs with fewer meats and fats. "Skip the bacon and eggs and have a healthy bowl of high-carb cereal with skim milk instead." The food pyramid exists primarily to decrease your fat intake—at the expense of your metabolic health.

Research confirms the food pyramid doesn't make us healthy. For example, the University of North Carolina at Chapel Hill's Gillings School of Global Public Health surveyed 8,721 Americans. Their study revealed a shocking 88 percent have poor metabolic health.[14] The food pyramid's guidelines, which the vast majority of Americans follow, has made most of us metabolically unhealthy.

MYTH #3: "THE FOOD PYRAMID IS BASED ON GOOD SCIENCE."

Most people who learn that the food pyramid is killing us ask something like, "How can this be? Isn't the food pyramid scientifically sound? The government uses the best studies to design it for us!"

As you'd hope, the food pyramid is studied and revised every five years by a committee.[15] The members of the committee are mostly scientists, but they have deep ties to the food industry. Researchers and clinicians

---

12 Jeff S. Volek and Richard D. Feinman, "Carbohydrate Restriction Improves the Features of Metabolic Syndrome. Metabolic Syndrome May be Defined by the Response to Carbohydrate Restriction," *Nutrition and Metabolism* 2 (2005). https://doi.org/10.1186/1743-7075-2-31.

13 Sunmin Park, Jaeouk Ahn, Nam-Soo Kim, Byung-Kook Lee, "High Carbohydrate Diets Are Positively Associated with the Risk of Metabolic Syndrome Irrespective to Fatty Acid Composition in Women: The KNHANES 2007-2014," *International Journal of Food Sciences and Nutrition* 68, no. 4 (2017): 479-487. https://doi.org/10.1080/09637486.2016.1252318.

14 "Only 12 percent of American Adults Are Metabolically Healthy, Carolina Study Finds," UNC Gillings School of Global Public Health, The University of North Carolina at Chapel Hill, last updated November 28, 2018, https://www.unc.edu/posts/2018/11/28/only-12-percent-of-american-adults-are-metabolically-healthy-carolina-study-finds/.

15 "Who's On the Guidelines Committee?" The Nutrition Coalition, last updated March 6, 2019, https://www.nutritioncoalition.us/news/2020-dietary-guidelines-committee.

get to raise their concerns, but the committee ultimately decides how to handle them.

At the risk of sounding cynical, I believe that many studies that would hurt committee members' stock portfolios get torpedoed. Science is applied selectively at best to the food pyramid. For more information on this ugly process, check out Nina Teicholz's books, as she delves into the medical and nutritional nightmare hidden behind the food pyramid guidelines.

Which brings us to our next myth . . .

MYTH #4: "THE PEOPLE WHO PRODUCE OUR FOOD WANT US TO BE HEALTHY."

Big Food is big business. The people who produce our food (and revise the food pyramid every five years) must create value for their shareholders by generating repeat customers.

Remember those 1990s Lay's chips commercials that ended with, "I bet you can't eat just one"? The executives of the company that used that slogan have a powerful influence over the committee setting the dietary guidelines for every American. This is a snapshot into the modern metabolic health epidemic.

The food industry is successful specifically because their food is unhealthy. The tobacco industry and sugar industry have borrowed each other's tactics. Even as early as the 1950s, research pointed at sugar as a serious heart health concern.[16,17] So the sugar industry hired scientists to "prove" the problem was really dietary fat.[18] Remember, the food pyramid was designed decades ago as a direct response to dietary fat being blamed

---

16 James Surowiecki, "A Big Tobacco Moment for the Sugar Industry," *New Yorker*, last updated September 15, 2016, https://www.newyorker.com/business/currency/a-big-tobacco-moment-for-the-sugar-industry.

17 Cristin E. Kearns, Laura A. Schmidt, Stanton A. Glantz, "Sugar Industry and Coronary Heart Disease Research: A Historical Analysis of Internal Industry Documents," *JAMA Internal Medicine* 176, no. 11 (2016): 1680-1685. https:// doi.org/ 10.1001/jamainternmed.2016.5394.

18 Camila Domonoske, "50 Years Ago, Sugar Industry Quietly Paid Scientists to Point Blame At Fat," The Two-Way, NPR, last updated September 13, 2016, https://www.npr.org/sections/thetwo-way/2016/09/13/493739074/50-years-ago-sugar-industry-quietly-paid-scientists-to-point-blame-at-fat.

for poor metabolic health. The corruption, in my opinion, could not be more obvious.

For most Americans, the sweet tooth addiction cycle begins the moment we eat solid food. Baby food is processed with simple carbohydrates and simple sugars. If the food industry gets you hooked early enough, they know they'll have a customer for life.

How does the food industry get away with this? They justify their manipulations by basically saying, "It's what the consumer wants." People want processed simple sugars with artificial colors and flavors that make them feel good. It's an addiction, and the food industry is happy to feed it.

But what if you stopped drinking sweetened soda pop for a week and had a can of seltzer of the same flavor instead? After the horrendous withdrawal symptoms have passed, you won't miss it. You're probably addicted right now and you don't even know it. That's why you can't stop eating and drinking the things that are killing you. I'm going to enlighten you so you can break those addictions.

Now, this book isn't here to take down the entire food industry. Plenty of other authors have written about that. This book is here to help you break free from the lies you've been fed (literally) so you can improve your health.

MYTH #5: "LOW-CARB DIETS ARE BAD FOR YOUR HEART."

Remember Atkins? There's a commonly repeated story that Dr. Atkins, the creator of the low-carb, high-fat Atkins diet, died from heart disease.[19] He actually slipped on ice, hit his head, suffered a traumatic brain injury, and suffered multiple organ failure. Who do you think funds the articles and encourages the rumors claiming that Dr. Atkins's diet killed him?

---

19 N. R. Kleinfield, "Just What Killed the Diet Doctor, and What Keeps the Issue Alive," *New York Times*, last updated February 11, 2004, https://www.nytimes.com/2004/02/11/nyregion/just-what-killed-the-diet-doctor-and-what-keeps-the-issue-alive.htm.

I'm a heart surgeon, and I'm here to tell you that low-carb diets are not bad for your health. They're bad for food industry shareholders. Would it surprise you to learn that scientific studies actually show that the more carbohydrates and less saturated fat that you consume, the greater your risk is of developing heart disease?[20] Additionally, we know that insulin resistance and diabetes are contributing risk factors for developing heart disease.[21] We also know that low-carbohydrate diets improve, and in some cases reverse, insulin resistance and diabetes.[22] Therefore, it would make *no* sense to think that low-carbohydrate diets would increase your risk for developing heart disease.

Let's unpack this thinking for a moment. What have the USDA guidelines and the food industry led you to believe? That dietary fats, especially saturated fats, will clog your arteries with cholesterol and cause heart disease. You may be surprised to learn that no matter how many times this myth gets repeated, there are no scientific studies to support this assertion.

So let's talk about the cholesterol myth.

MYTH #6: "HIGH CHOLESTEROL CAUSES HEART DISEASE."

You've probably heard that the higher your LDL—often called the "bad" cholesterol—the higher your risk of heart disease. But about half the patients I operate on for coronary heart disease have low or normal LDL. Some are on medications, some are not. And there's data to suggest that

---

20 Teresa R. Haugsgjerd , Grace M. Egeland, Ottar K Nygård, Jannicke Igland, Gerhard Sulo, Vegard Lysne, Kathrine J. Vinknes, Kjetil Bjornevik, and Grethe S. Tel, "Intake of Carbohydrates and SFA and Risk of CHD in Middle-Age Adults: the Hordaland Health Study (HUSK)," *Public Health Nutrition* (2020): 1-15. https:// doi.org/ 10.1017/S1368980020003043.
21 Valeska Ormazabal, Soumyalekshmi Nair, Omar Elfeky, Claudio Aguayo, Carlos Salomon, and Felipe A. Zuñiga, "Association between Insulin Resistance and the Development of Cardiovascular Disease," *Cardiovascular Diabetology* 17, no. 122 (2018). https://doi.org/10.1186/s12933-018-0762-4.
22 Mary Caffrey, "After a Year, Low-Carb Diet Helps Many Patients Reverse Type 2 Diabetes, Lose Weight, and Stop Insulin," AJMC, last updated February 12, 2018, https://www.ajmc.com/view/after-a-year-low-carb-diet-helps-many-patients-reverse-type-2-diabetes-lose-weight-and-stop-insulin.

half of people with ideal cholesterol levels still have a risk of developing heart problems.[23]

Sure, cholesterol plays a part in heart disease, but it is not the single cause we've been led to believe. Based on my experience, HDL and triglycerides are more predictive of heart disease than LDL. We only focus on LDL because that's the cholesterol physicians can easily manipulate with medications. In fact, research indicates that in the setting of good metabolic health, the higher the HDL, the longer you can expect to live.[24] When I teach my patients about cholesterol, they're shocked. If you're ready to be shocked, too, here's how it actually works:

Once you have poor metabolic health, your blood vessels become inflamed. The body then sends cholesterol as a repair mechanism to try and fix that inflammation. Imagine repairing an old, crumbling wall with some spackle. Cholesterol is the spackle your body smears on your blood vessels to keep them intact. And if the wall keeps getting damaged and you keep piling on the spackle, eventually you'll start to block up the blood vessel. But the problem isn't the cholesterol; it's the inflamed blood vessels and the damage being done that necessitates the cholesterol!

This is why the concept of cholesterol as the main problem never sat well with me. The assumption is that cholesterol is basically a poison your body produces that kills you. In fact, it's only trying to fix other issues created by the foods you are eating. So the answer is obviously not to attack the spackling on the wall, but to stop damaging your walls in the first place.

Cholesterol isn't the cause of heart disease. Poor metabolic health is.

---

23 "Half of Patients with Ideal Cholesterol Have Underlying Heart Risks," CardioSmart, American College of Cardiology, last updated December 14, 2017, https://www.cardiosmart.org/news/2017/12/half-of-patients-with-ideal-cholesterol-have-underlying-heart-risks.

24 Fredrick Kunkle, "Gene for HDL Cholesterol Linked to Longer Life, Study Finds," *Washington Post*, last updated November 7, 2014, https://www.washingtonpost.com/national/health-science/gene-for-hdl-cholesterol-linked-to-longer-life-study-finds/2014/11/07/f277c16e-6628-11e4-9fdc-d43b053ecb4d_story.html.

MYTH #7: "MEDICATIONS ARE THE BEST TREATMENT FOR MEDICAL ISSUES."

Many doctors are quick to throw medication at a problem to treat symptoms and slow to discuss lifestyle and diet changes to address the underlying causes. Partly to blame is the assumption that these problems are genetic or just plain unknowable. But as you've seen, that's not usually true. Metabolic health is the issue. Therefore, medications that only treat the symptoms are not the best treatment. They exist to alleviate symptoms and keep the patient alive while the real causes are addressed. They are *not* a long-term solution.

In my experience, many doctors assume people aren't willing to change their diet. That's untrue from my perspective. Most people can follow dietary guidelines. Because they already do. The food pyramid is effective at snaring food industry customers precisely because so many people try to follow it. But doctors perceive that their patients don't follow advice because the patients don't get better. The real issue is that the advice itself is flawed. "Eat low fat and count your calories" is not sound advice to improve metabolic health.

If the advice works, my experience is that people will enthusiastically follow it. People don't want to be unhealthy and miserable. If there was a magical diet that made you drop a hundred pounds and keep it off, everyone in America would start that diet today. (There is, sort of, but it's not a pill or waist band. It's a system. More on that system soon.)

Another severe problem is that pharmaceutical companies have tremendous influence over the medical industry, beginning with medical school involvement. The healthcare industry is built for business. Hospitals need patients. And pharmaceutical companies need repeat customers. So the education system teaches doctors to pile up medications to treat every symptom, then treat side effects with more meds.

It's also quicker for an overworked doctor to write a prescription and rush out the door than to communicate the message of this book inside a tiny office visit.

Yet there is no example I'm aware of that treating a disease is as effective as not having the disease in the first place. Stopping your patients from getting sick in the first place is the very best medicine. It's every doctor's dream, but few know how to achieve it. The tools to do so have been withheld from us in favor of the repeat customer model.

So, am I saying you should just follow a metabolically healthy diet, eat this and not that, and everything will be perfect? Not exactly . . .

MYTH #8: "DIETS WORK IF YOU FOLLOW THEM."

Is this a myth? Who knows? People stop following diets because they're too hard to follow.

Most diet plans have you do things that are not sustainable. Sure, you might quickly lose weight like I did when I was in my twenties, but that's the business model. They know you'll be back. Because once you come off these impossible restrictions, you'll pack the weight right back on. If you've been conditioned from birth to be addicted to sugar and processed food, it's going to take more than a month of crash dieting to undo the conditioning that keeps you unhealthy.

By the way, that's exactly why I don't give you a fad diet to follow in this book. I teach you sustainable lifestyle changes you can maintain for *the rest of your life*. If you're successful on my program, you shouldn't need me anymore. Unlike other authors, I don't want repeat customers. I'm just trying to keep you off my surgery table so I don't watch you die.

I work with people directly for one year, they see the results, and the results stick. I see other people doing one fad diet after another over and over while taking medications for five, ten, or fifteen years. Medications are a subscription product. Big Pharma is not in the business of selling you products that you soon won't need anymore.

Dietary changes don't have to be hard. What's hard is the "you just have to hunker down for thirty days" mentality that teaches you to crave sugars and processed foods even more than before. You think of *nothing else* for those thirty days! Real, sustainable dietary changes don't make you miserable. You can eat in a way that makes you feel satisfied, not hungry, and not ridden with cravings, and you still get healthy.

The truth is that there is not one ideal human diet. One diet cannot fit every person. There is no one right diet out there. Nothing on the market is guaranteed to help you, even for thirty days.

There may be an ideal human diet, ancestrally speaking. We all essentially ate the same diet as we evolved. Food variety is unique to humans. Out in the wild, animals choose three to four foods they specialize in finding. Prior to the period ten thousand to fifty thousand years ago, humans were the same: we had no variety. We ate what was available where we lived.

The problem today is, everyone comes from a different place. Even when we try to eat healthy, we've got an entire grocery store full of options that our ancestors never had, and some of our ancestral dietary requirements differ. That means the food one person needs may not be right for the next person. Look at the way doctors prescribe medications: each individual person has different needs, and their needs change over time. The same is true of dietary choices. What I offer you in this book is not a diet. It's science-based, sustainable lifestyle changes to improve your metabolic health—and your entire life.

MYTH #9: "TRYING TO LOSE WEIGHT BY RESTRICTING CALORIES ALWAYS WORKS."

What most diet plans have in common is some attempt to restrict calories. The almost universal diet advice is, "Eat less than you need to create a calorie deficit. This will make you burn fat."

But caloric surplus and deficit measurements are based on guesswork. We don't have an accurate way of knowing how many calories we're eating and burning. Even mainstream medicine, for all their foibles, admits that accurate calorie burn calculation is "difficult."[25] We can guesstimate. That's about it. A person with more muscle mass may burn more calories doing the same activity as someone with half their musculature, or someone of a different age or sex. When you eat more protein, your metabolic rate will increase, so if you eat a low amount of calories with higher protein, you'll be burning more than someone with a lower protein intake and the same amount of calories.

What we do know is the type of calories you eat goes a long way in determining how much weight you lose.[26] Not all calories are created (or consumed) equal.

MYTH #10: "THE BEST WAY TO BURN CALORIES IS EXERCISE."

The data shows you can't out-exercise a bad diet. Metabolic health is 90 percent diet, 10 percent lifestyle, and exercise is *not* necessary for weight loss.

In fact, exercise itself might cause you to violate your dietary changes. The more you exercise, the hungrier you get. Forty-five minutes of intense working out only burns 200–300 calories but makes you so hungry that you stop on the way home from the gym and consume an 800-calorie burger. Even snacking on a nutrition bar might bring in an average of 220 calories. That means your entire workout only burned the food you ate as a result of working out. And exercise doesn't necessarily access the fat stores you want to lose.

---

25 Kellie Bramlet Blackburn, "How to Determine Calorie Burn," MD Anderson Cancer Center, last updated June 2017, https://www.mdanderson.org/publications/focused-on-health/How-to-determine-calorie-burn. h27Z1591413.html.
26 Celia Smoak Spell, "There's No Sugar-Coating It: All Calories Are Not Created Equal," Harvard Health Blog, Harvard Medical School, last updated November 4, 2016, https://www.health.harvard.edu/blog/theres-no-sugar-coating-it-all-calories-are-not-created-equal-2016110410602.

I'm not telling you not to exercise. Physical activity has a whole range of health benefits that bring you energy, give your body flexibility, and make you happier overall. Instead of focused activity that increases your hunger, a better plan is to build consistent movement into your entire day. Moving your body throughout the day is just as effective as working out for most people.

MYTH #11: "YOU CAN'T IMPROVE METABOLIC HEALTH CONDITIONS WITHOUT MEDICATION."

Not only is this statement purely false, it creates hopelessness and the dangerous belief that people should just give up on their health. That fuels a perpetual cycle that ends on my surgical table.

Have you ever heard a doctor say that you can get off medications for chronic conditions like diabetes or high blood pressure? My clients have gotten off these medications. Type 2 diabetes is reversible, based on both studies and my personal experience with patients. You can also improve your blood pressure without medication, also based on both research and my personal experience.[27]

The medications are there to treat the symptoms. That means the meds will never make you better, they just prevent you from getting worse as fast as you would without them. Eventually your problems will still catch up with you if you don't address the underlying causes for the symptoms.

MYTH #12: "HEALTH PROBLEMS COME WITH AGE."

This might be the saddest myth of all—that we're supposed to get sicker and weaker as we age, beginning in our fifties and sixties, and should expect decades of miserable decline as we lose out on family events and personal pleasure.

---

27 "Low-Carb Diet Effective at Lowering Blood Pressure," ScienceDaily, last updated January 26, 2010, https://www.sciencedaily.com/releases/2010/01/100125172938.htm.

This is deeply wrong. You can live healthy your whole life and die in your nineties. We shouldn't have a ten- to twenty-year period of our lives where we're progressively dying day by day and miserable the whole time.

One example of this lie is the belief that hormonal imbalance is the natural result of aging and that nothing can be done about it apart from medication. For example, some claim that testosterone naturally decreases with age. No, low T is more closely associated with poor metabolic health.[28] That's why healthy men in their eighties can have even more testosterone than obese men in their twenties. It's all about how you fuel your body.

People also assume female hormones naturally destabilize with age. The dreaded menopause is held up as a life-shattering event that could tear apart your whole world for years on end. But many women improve some menopausal symptoms by going on low-carb, whole-food diets.[29]

Your body isn't designed to just fall apart from your thirties onward. Don't let anyone make you believe this.

SO, WHERE DID ALL THESE MYTHS COME FROM?

These are just the twelve biggest lies that pertain to our conversation here in this book. There are so many other deceptions and half-truths buried in the medical and food industries if you go digging.

It can seem overwhelming to learn there are so many outright lies that have intentionally infected the public's health as well as medical practitioners' knowledge and advice. Doctors at least should have the truth, right? People die because of these myths!

When my patients learn about these lies, they demand answers. "How did we get here? How can our whole medical system be teaching wrong information? And what can I do to protect myself?"

---

28 Vakkat Muraleedharan and T. Hugh Jones, "Testosterone and the metabolic syndrome," Therapeutic Advances in Endocrinology and Metabolism 1, no. 5 (2010): 207-223. https://doi.org/10.1177/2042018810390258.
29 Rachael Link and Alyssa Northrop, "Can the Keto Diet Help with Menopause?" Healthline, last updated August 28, 2020, https://www.healthline.com/nutrition/keto-and-menopause.

I'm going to help you discover these answers and discover that you can be healthy and thriving. And while I may not have all the answers (no one does), I can help you establish a framework based on the relentless pursuit of good health and how to evaluate the information you hear regarding how to be healthy. And first, let's discuss how we as a culture got to a place where these myths are pervasive and accepted as gospel truth—and what you can do about it.

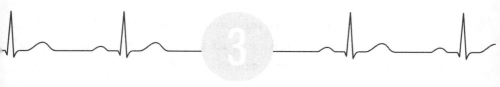

THE SYSTEM IS BROKEN
(AND WHAT TO DO ABOUT IT)

"This can't be right." I tapped the computer screen to show the nurse. "How can his blood sugar numbers be this high?"

She glanced at Alex's chart and cringed. "I'm not sure. But that's not good. He's still recovering from his coronary artery bypass . . ."

"Right, but there's no way his numbers should be this bad. I'll go talk to him."

As I walked down the hall to my patient's room, I racked my brain trying to figure out what could be causing the issue. A medication he hadn't disclosed? Prediabetic symptoms we hadn't caught? What else could it be?

I knocked lightly on Alex's open door before walking in. "Morning, Alex, it's Dr. Ova—" My breath stuck in my throat.

There was my patient, propped up in bed, with his breakfast tray in front of him. Pancakes with low-fat syrup, low-fat yogurt with granola, a cup of sweetened peaches, a small sausage patty, a small serving of scrambled eggs (likely artificial egg substitute), and a cup of orange juice.

Well, that explains the blood sugar, I thought. A cursory assessment of his breakfast told me he was eating at least 700 calories, 40 to 50 percent of which came straight from carbs. And this was the lowest-carb breakfast I could have ordered for Alex. Sure, the assortment was in line with the food pyramid and low in fat, but it was still excessive—even dangerous to Alex's recovery. Eating sweet, processed carbohydrates in this quantity after a heart bypass is like smoking a pack a day after lung cancer surgery. It doesn't make any sense. Hospitals *have* to offer better food than this. But, of course, many can't.

Hospitals must serve low-fat, high-carb meals like Alex's breakfast due to dietary guidelines. Following the rules is a prerequisite to getting paid by Medicare and private insurance. But eating like this leads many people right back to the hospital. A system that incentivizes this is clearly broken. Here's how we got here.

HOW THE MEDICAL SYSTEM ACTUALLY WORKS

Metabolic health is the core of my message. I believe that's what will keep people off my operating table. I'll educate everyone I can about it. And to do that, I need to confront the observations I've made as a physician.

Something has gone wrong in the healthcare system. We've lost sight of preventing people from getting disease, and we're focused on just treating the diseases once people have them. For most physicians, it's not even a thought that we can prevent chronic conditions like diabetes and heart disease. And we're told they're permanent, that we can't undo the damage. We as doctors are taught that it's normal to be on multiple medications when you're fifty years old.

Meanwhile, most medical professionals are not properly educated about your nutritional needs.[30] The average doctor and nutritionist is unaware of the data you've already taken from this book. Those who do educate themselves and discover the problems in the current dietary guidelines are afraid to buck the system. Consider the financial incentive as well: many hospitals and clinics are forced to follow government guidelines in order to get paid.

---

30 Rachel Cernansky, "Your Doctor May Not be the Best Source of Nutrition Advice," *Washington Post*, last updated July 8, 2018, https://www.washingtonpost.com/national/health-science/your-doctor-may-not-be-the-best-source-of-nutrition-advice/2018/07/06/f8b3ecfe-78af-11e8-93cc-6d3beccdd7a3_story.html.

Compensation itself is built around disease treatment, not prevention. Food companies, pharmaceutical companies, and their involvement in medical education build the system around the often expensive and usually recurring treatment of disease. Everything relies on those institutions' funding and guidance. The entire system would break if we shifted priorities from treatment to prevention.

The family doctor or primary care physician is supposed to prevent the medical issues, but they've got student loans to pay and need to support their families and pay their staff. If they have a patient with high blood pressure or high cholesterol, the doctor's compensation is partially dependent on meeting guidelines that are mostly focused on prescribing medicines. Although guidelines are directly related to health, nutrition recommendations are not a check box for compensation. If you want to get paid, look at the prescription list first.

I do believe that the vast majority of physicians are not malicious and genuinely try to put their patients first. But some scientists and past thought leaders have been intentional about self-promotion over the greater good. Much of the science that led to the current nutritional guidelines was poorly done.

Now add to this situation a general shortage of physicians, which has resulted in a decreased average time healthcare providers spend with each patient. Doctors who do become aware of the nutritional guideline deficiencies don't really have time to discuss them with their patients. Discussing lifestyle choices, metabolism, and the impact food has on our health may save lives, but with just fifteen minutes per patient, most physicians opt for the quickest fix and skip right to medicine.

Some doctors may tell themselves that medication buys the patient time to research food on their own. But with the entire medical system telling patients to follow the food pyramid, the reality is that medication just buys time before those patients end up on my operating table.

There's also a generational issue at play here. A hundred years ago, before rapid transit and international food trades were possible, people ate what was available. Even our grandparents and great-grandparents were eating whole food because processed food wasn't affordable. But the booming population led to an increase in processed foods, which brought new health issues.

Our parents' generations realized there was some connection between diet and health, but they weren't sure what it was. We already discussed the deception from the sugar industry in constructing the food pyramid. When those guidelines got pushed on our parents' generation, they assumed the guidelines were right—because who could imagine the medical system would be complicit in harming people?

This is why we've seen various crusades against certain types of foods, then paradoxical pendulum swings as the "experts" decide they got it wrong—but this time they're sure! Our parents were told low-fat foods with vegetable oils would save their lives, so they threw out the animal-based butter and smeared margarine on everything. And when this has failed to improve our health, they claim that people aren't following their advice and continue to push for even lower-fat diets. They targeted eggs the same way—cholesterol causes heart disease, and eggs have cholesterol, so don't eat eggs. Then came the push for more dairy ("Got Milk?"), but experts questioned that idea because whole and 2 percent milk contain fat. Switch to skim milk. And while you're at it, set down the regular soda and pick up a lower-calorie alternative with all its artificial colors, flavors, and sweeteners. With each diet fad and nutritional guideline updates, the root issue—metabolic health—has yet to improve.

My personal view of the healthcare industry is colored by my experience both as a care provider and as an individual who struggled with poor metabolic health and its consequences. I've spent my career dealing with the end result of not addressing metabolic health. Patients failed by the medical system end up on my surgical table, often when it's too late. I became a surgeon to help heal people's hearts, not to watch them die.

I didn't recognize the system was wrong until I learned the truth about metabolic health. I'd been taught the standard lie in medical school: cholesterol and saturated fat cause heart disease, so take your statins. In my experience, all twelve myths in the previous chapter are taught to doctors as *truth*. When I learned the truth and witnessed the changes in my own life, I realized these "facts" were wrong.

What bothered me most of all was the heart disease patients who were not obese and had low cholesterol and no genetic history of heart disease. Yet in they came with heart issues anyway. According to the current medical model, that shouldn't be happening. It was only when I realized these patients were still metabolically unhealthy—skinny fat—that the pieces clicked into place. They faced the same issues as my obese patients because they were struggling with the same problems. Only their outward manifestations were different.

My current worldview crystallized completely when I learned that while cholesterol does play a part in the disease process, dietary cholesterol consumption is not an inciting event.[31] That flies in the face of every modern medical belief. High cholesterol with metabolic wellness is not the problem we've been told it is. We are treating the wrong problem and leaving patients to die while they believe they're being saved.

I remember as a surgeon realizing for the first time that I was being paid to oversee the tail end of a deadly system. I had lunch with a colleague and told him, "If only these people were educated about what I now know, they could have prevented these problems, and my services would be needed a lot less." He looked confused and asked, "Are you trying to put yourself out of business?"

---

31 Ann Pietrangelo, "Does High Cholesterol Cause Heart Disease?" Healthline, last updated March 16, 2020, https://www.healthline.com/health/cholesterol-and-heart-disease.

It's still horrifying to me that hospitals serve the same foods that put you there in the first place. Ninety percent of the food we serve follows the high-carb, low-fat, "heart-healthy" diet. And yet, most people who need heart surgery are diabetic or prediabetic. We often have insulin in an IV during and after heart surgery so that we have better outcomes because the patient's body can barely function on their current diet.

I think often about that first conversation with my colleague. "Are you trying to put yourself out of business?" The answer is yes. I gave an interview recently, and the interviewer asked me the same thing. "Doesn't your metabolic education threaten your surgery paycheck? If everyone gets healthy, you'll be out of a job."

The answer I gave then is the same one I'll tell you now. "That's exactly what I want. I'm a horrible businessman because I'm looking to put myself out of business."

If everyone gets healthy, and I have to pivot my nutrition clinic into full-time mode, I'd be thrilled. Because I'd know I saved lives. And that's why I became a doctor in the first place.

That's also why my consultations run longer than a typical physician's fifteen-minute chat. I know that medication isn't going to keep my patients off the table a second time. Only dietary education and lifestyle changes can help. I believe in this so much that I even spend time off the clock when I'm not being paid to consult with patients I know will die without this lifesaving truth. People need to know, and it's my sacred duty to care for them. The oath I took as a doctor demands I teach the truth to people who will die without it.

As a surgeon, while I'm doing necessary and helpful work, I know I can address patient health needs before they require surgery. I couldn't live with myself if I didn't do something about that. Other physicians have felt the same, and I'm enormously grateful to the medical providers who have stepped up to spread this information. Without them, I never would have had access to the information that changed my life, that allowed me to become healthy, and that now allows me to save the lives of patients who rely on me.

Even so, physicians have been persecuted for offering counter-industry advice. Tim Noakes in South Africa and Gary Fettke in Australia were each brought up on charges related to giving nonstandard advice on metabolic health. Both fought the medical industry, who could not let their alternate diet advice slide. Both were ultimately cleared of wrongdoing, and Dr. Fettke eventually received an apology from regulators, but the pushback from the healthcare system and the processed-food industry served as a warning to anyone who might dare to step out of line.

Despite the warning, the career risk, and the system pushback, I continue to believe it's worth it to share these nutritional truths. I'll do anything I can to keep patients off my operating table. I don't want to witness even one more preventable death. That includes yours. I hope you'll take the next section of the book to heart and do your own research as you discover what your body needs to stay alive and thrive in your golden years.

IT'S TIME TO SAVE YOUR LIFE

I've got a challenge for you.

I made the bold step of switching from treating to preventing disease. I've put my professional paycheck on the line. I also applied all the lessons in this book to my own life. Everything you're going to read in the pages ahead are sustainable changes I live by every day. They saved my life. They've saved the lives of patients and coaching clients I've worked with over the years. And they'll save your life, too, if you're willing to commit to this program.

Are you ready to commit? You've learned about the system working against you. You know your life's on the line. Are you willing to give this change a chance and see your metabolic health improve?

If you're still reading, you're declaring that enough is enough. It's time to change.

Good. It's time to talk logistics. Let's discuss exactly how you're going to change your metabolic health forever and live the kind of life the medical system tells you is impossible without prescription drugs.

HOW TO MEASURE, ASSESS, AND IMPROVE YOUR METABOLIC HEALTH

"What do you mean, I'm . . . 'metabolically unhealthy?'" my new client Jack asked. "My family doctor says I'm fine. I'm only on two medications. One for my blood pressure, one statin for my LDL."

A mutual friend had referred Jack to my nutrition practice because he had been feeling low energy. His intake form listed high blood pressure and high LDL cholesterol, but he figured his two prescriptions made those a nonissue.

I had to give Jack the bad news. When lies have been programmed into your mindset your whole life, the first step is to hear the truth—even if it's hard to hear.

I held up Jack's blood panel results for him to see. "You did these blood tests with your doctor. We'll go through them together and check the five metabolic health signs I look for."

Metabolic health is indicated by five specific markers. We all fail the metabolic health test if three or more of these markers are off. Again, 88 percent of Americans are currently failing at least one of the metabolic health markers, and most don't even realize it. Many end up on an operating table. Now that I actively work to keep people off mine, they're the sort of people I help in my metabolic consulting practice.

I laid Jack's test results on my desk. "First, go ahead and stand up, please. Let's measure your waist."

"Oh, my pants size is—"

"Pants size isn't the marker, Jack. We need your waist circumference just above your belly button."

"But my doctor says my weight is perfect."

"Your weight may be fine, but weight is a poor indicator for health. We need to measure your waist instead. For women, we look for thirty-five inches or fewer. For men, forty inches or fewer. Anything above that indicates an 80 percent chance of metabolic syndrome."

Jack stood up silently, and I measured his waist.

"Thirty-eight inches. Good news, you're under the cutoff. Now, let's look at these blood panel results."

Jack sat back down, but he eyed the paperwork suspiciously. "I always thought that weight was everything."

"No, and you'll see why." I pointed to a line on his test results. "See this number here, your fasting blood glucose level? It's 120. Healthy is less than 100 mg per deciliter. Most people, unfortunately, run around 110, which isn't diabetic, but it's reaching prediabetic. Full diabetic is 125."

"Well, my doctor said I'm not diabetic."

"That's right, technically you're not. But a fasting blood glucose level above 100 is the second marker for metabolic syndrome. Blood pressure is the third. For good metabolic health, your top number should be less than 130 and your bottom number less than 85 without medication."

"Blood pressure? No way. Everybody has high blood pressure. It's just part of getting older."

"It is when you live in a culture with food and stress like ours. But it's not medically normal for an entire population to develop blood pressure problems with age. In some cases, there is a reason to have high blood pressure from rare causes like tumors. Otherwise, it is commonly called essential hypertension, and this is an indicator of poor metabolic health. It's not about age, it's about the amount of time on a metabolically unhealthy diet."

"Aha," Jack said with a smile. "I've got you there. I'm already on a low-sodium diet."

"Salt has very little if anything to do with high blood pressure. New data show that a high-saline IV actually lowers blood pressure.[32] Here's the problem: Lower salt foods taste bland. Often, adding sugar results in a better taste. Even to dishes with meat and vegetables. Junk food is loaded with sugar, salt, and fat. The old assumption is that salt results in high blood pressure, but it's actually the processed food the salt is in and all the sugar loaded in for flavor."

"You gotta be kidding me. Everyone knows salt is bad for you. Right?"

"Actually, I put sea salt in my coffee and on my meats. Most of us are mineral deficient. In my experience, that's from not eating enough quality salt. Unrefined sea salt, like Celtic or Himalayan, that is, not white table salt." I paused. "OK, the fourth marker of metabolic health. That's going to be your HDL cholesterol. For men, a 'bad' HDL number is less than forty, for women it's less than fifty."

"Well, I'm on a statin for my cholesterol. So that should already be helping."

"That's your LDL cholesterol, which isn't the issue. Doctors labeled LDL as 'bad' cholesterol as soon as statins were released. But statins were a solution without a problem—a product without a use. So advertisers created one. The function of all cholesterol is to transport fats around your body as an energy source. They play a part in immune function and cell membranes. We actually want HDL to be high."

Jack still looked skeptical. "High cholesterol? That's opposite from what I've always heard. Are you sure?"

---

32 Tim Newman, "High Blood Pressure: Sodium May Not Be the Culprit," Medical News Today, last updated April 25, 2017, https://www.medicalnewstoday.com/articles/317099.

"Yes. Normally a family doctor only looks at LDL, but HDL and triglycerides are better indicators of health. With triglycerides, the fifth marker, you do want less than 150. Triglycerides transport fat back and forth between your intestines, liver, and bloodstream." I pointed to another line on his test results. "Yours are high, and that means your body is working overtime to transport the fat."

I set down Jack's blood panel results and looked him in the eye. "Jack, you're not obese, but your body is acting as though you are. You meet four of the criteria for metabolic syndrome—high blood glucose, high blood pressure, high triglycerides, and low HDL cholesterol. Metabolic issues are the cause. Prescription medications only treat the symptoms. And if you don't solve the underlying problem, it can kill you."

Jack sat back in his chair and blew out a sigh. "I don't know what to say. My doctor said I'm fine, I just have a couple of problems. I take my meds like I'm supposed to. But you make it sound like I have worse problems, and my meds are just covering them up. You're scaring me here. What should I do?"

....

Most people who come into my office or those with whom I have a telemedicine visit have no clue how to measure their health. They rely on doctors to warn them when they stray into the danger zone. But that only allows for emergency treatment once a person progresses to such poor metabolic health that they're at risk of severe, life-threatening problems.

Notice that LDL is not an indicator of metabolic health. But doctors are often quick to throw a patient on a statin and assume that will prevent them from getting heart disease and extend their life. Meanwhile, the pharmaceutical industry has also tried to go after HDL, but medications developed to raise HDL have failed. And the truth is that we don't need them!

Research shows if you have a high HDL and low triglycerides, you can expect a longer lifetime.[33,34] In my experience, this counts even if you have high LDL. But the vast majority of heart patients I've had to operate on have had low HDL and high triglycerides. That combination is a disaster for your long-term health. So how do we flip our HDL and triglycerides without medication?

People are being educated in the opposite direction from where they need to go. And they imagine that as long as they're not obese, they're fine. To fix these misconceptions and lies, I'm going to teach you all about the real markers of metabolic health and how to measure them. Then in Part II and Part III of this book, you'll learn how to fix them.

THE FIVE MARKERS OF METABOLIC HEALTH

As I told Jack, the criteria for diagnosing metabolic syndrome are:

1. Waist circumference over 35 inches for women, and over 40 inches for men
2. Fasting blood glucose of 100 mg/dl or greater or taking glucose-lowering medications
3. Blood pressure higher than 130/85 mm Hg or taking blood-pressure-lowering medications
4. HDL cholesterol less than 40 mg/dL for men or 50 mg/dL for women
5. Triglycerides over 150 mg/dL

33 Jian Wang, Liwei Shi, Yunfeng Zou, Jiexia Tang, Jiansheng Cai, Yi Wei, Jian Qin, and Zhiyong Zhang, "Positive association of familial longevity with the moderate-high HDL-C concentration in Bama Aging Study," *Aging* 10, no. 11 (2018): 3528-3540. https://doi.org/10.18632/aging.101663.
34 Anika A. M. Vaarhorst, Marian Beekman, Eka H. D. Suchiman, Diana van Heemst, Jeanine J. Houwing-Duistermaat, Rudi G. J. Westendorp, P. Eline Slagboom, Bastiaan T. Heijmans, Leiden Longevity Study (LLS) Group, "Lipid metabolism in long-lived families: The Leiden Longevity Study," *AGE* 33 (2011): 219-227. https://doi.org/10.1007/s11357-010-9172-6.

Having three of the five criteria establishes the diagnosis of metabolic syndrome; however, even having one or two of these criteria is a warning sign of having poor metabolic health.

The single most predictive sign is waist circumference, which is why we associate obesity with metabolic health. It's almost impossible to see the other four markers from the outside, after all. But they all matter, because a person can avoid obesity and still fail the other four criteria.

There's a saying that goes, "You can only manage what you can measure." It's absolutely true. But most people have no idea what their health numbers are because they don't know how to interpret the results. Many clients who come into my office have never had a blood panel done.

Even having normal blood glucose can be misleading. A lot of people have normal blood glucose but very high insulin. That means the body is making an excessive amount of insulin to deal with the excess carbs the person is eating. Over the years, the body becomes less sensitive to insulin. Eventually, blood glucose goes up, but insulin levels can be too high for up to ten years before that's reflected in glucose levels. This is why testing insulin levels is better, as it can be incredibly helpful in determining metabolic health. We often start with blood glucose because that test is simpler to order and has often already been tested when clients come to me. But if glucose is under 100, I order an insulin test as a more accurate measurement to be sure. Most healthcare professionals tell you that insulin of less than 20 is the target, but I tell people less than 10 is ideal.

There are obese people who meet none of the criteria and are metabolically healthy, but that is exceedingly rare. You can be obese and still have acceptable blood pressure and glucose. This usually happens among younger people before the full effects of a bad diet catch up with them.

As an overweight young man, I probably had a couple of these that were OK. I know what it's like to tell yourself, "It's OK, I only have one or two, it's no big deal." It was a shock for me to discover I was far more metabolically unhealthy than I ever realized.

One question I get a lot is, "What about sumo wrestlers?" And that's a worthwhile question, because they're held up as some of the fattest people on earth. They consume a mountain of carbs and salts. But the truth is that their body contains vast muscle mass. Where they should be metabolically unhealthy, their dense muscle system compensates. Now, as they get older and their intense physical training and wrestling decreases, if they don't change their diet they do become metabolically unhealthy. But at the peak of their game, sumo wrestlers are healthier than most Americans.

Which brings me to a major point: I don't care if you're obese. I care if you're metabolically unhealthy because that lands people on my operating table. I commonly operate on people who are not obese, but it is rare that I operate on a metabolically healthy person. My goal isn't to create a nation of skinny people who look like Hollywood superstars. As I mentioned before, you can also be in a healthy weight range but be metabolically unhealthy. You could be thinner than I am but have worse health. Weight doesn't matter. Metabolic health matters. It doesn't matter to me what you look like on the outside. I just want you to live a long life with maximum energy and minimal pain.

To get you there, I need to teach you how to measure your real markers of metabolic health.

MEASURE BEFORE YOU MANAGE: HOW TO MEASURE THE FIVE MARKERS

WAIST CIRCUMFERENCE

The best way to measure your waist is with a cloth tape measure. Measure in the morning before you eat so your food doesn't increase your reading.

Relax your stomach so you're not sucking it in. Wrap the tape measure around your bare stomach just above your belly button. Then draw the tape measure snug, but don't cinch down tight.

As I mentioned, the target number for women is under thirty-five inches, and it's under forty for men. That doesn't change as you age, as long as you're over eighteen years old. If you're very short or very tall, a more specific ideal number for optimum metabolic health is less than half of your height.

BLOOD PRESSURE

Checking your blood pressure is easier than ever these days. You can go to your doctor and get it done, but you can also stop by most pharmacies where they have a blood pressure machine out front for customer use. If you'd rather do it in your home, you can buy electronic blood pressure cuffs in stores or online with easy instructions.

Make sure that you check your blood pressure at different times, including morning, midday, and evening. And some people get nervous seeing their doctor, or even the first time they use a blood pressure machine, so checking multiple times lets you know where your real levels are apart from stress. Ideally you're looking for blood pressure 130/85 or lower.

EVERYTHING ELSE

Fasting Blood Glucose, Insulin, HDL Cholesterol, and Triglycerides

All of these tests except insulin are part of annual blood panels. You can work with your doctor on getting these done as part of your routine care.

While it's not technically part of the five markers, I do recommend getting your fasting insulin level checked if possible. You're usually going to have to ask your doctor specifically to check this, and many doctors won't order the test because they honestly don't know what to do with it. If you're not diabetic, they won't want to worry about it. This is one reminder to start looking for a physician who is knowledgeable about metabolic health. Fortunately, there are some workaround options for people who don't have such a doctor yet.

The great news is that you can order your own blood work these days. The only states that don't allow this are New York, New Jersey, and Rhode

Island. Sites like **ownyourlabs.com** make it cheap and easy to check your own blood work without worrying about your doctor refusing specific tests.

If you get blood work ordered from a doctor, you may get charged a hundred dollars, insurance might only pay fifteen dollars, and your copay will be another fifteen dollars. But if you use a website, you could pay $8.75 for a test that cost the testing company even less than that. I recommend using the website, but go the route that makes the best sense for your needs and gives you confidence in your results.

Ideally, you're looking for blood glucose under 100, insulin under 10, HDL above 40 for men or 50 for women, and triglycerides under 150. A surrogate marker for insulin resistance, if you are unable to get your insulin level directly, is the ratio between triglycerides and your HDL level. If this ratio is less than 2, there is a good chance that you are not insulin resistant.

METABOLIC HEALTH MARKER MAINTENANCE

When clients who are metabolically unhealthy come to me, we re-check their blood work every three months until they reach their goals. Once they do, we recheck them every six to twelve months depending on their symptoms and overall health. I recommend reordering blood tests for yourself (or with your doctor) every three months until you achieve metabolic health as well.

I have clients measure their waistline weekly. This isn't to teach them to obsess over thinness, but because the waistline is the simplest measurement of metabolic issues. Plus, this test is free! Clients can track this progress over time to see fluctuations due to hormone changes or dietary variance. Fluctuation is normal, but gaining two inches and holding on to it could indicate a serious health change that may need to be addressed.

Continuous glucose monitoring is also key to tracking changes and being able to see the metabolic impact of exactly what you're eating and drinking. When someone starts tracking their metabolic health, I usually recommend they wear a glucose monitor for ten to fourteen days to track their blood sugar changes in real time. It even pairs up to your phone for easy use.

Following your blood sugar changes educates you on how your body reacts to what you're consuming, and it gives you a heads-up on issues right on the spot. But when people ask their doctors for a glucose monitor, most physicians say, "You're crazy! You don't need that, that's for diabetics!" I say, why wait for diabetes to hit? Why not look at which foods are spiking your blood sugar so you can be healthier *now*?

The unfortunate news is that it isn't easy to procure one of these glucose monitors. You do need a prescription for the ones currently on the market. I've heard rumors that a major tech company is working on a monitor you can wear on your wrist, but I haven't seen any announcements on that as of writing this book.

The good news is that there's nothing preventing any doctor from prescribing you one of these monitors. They may think you're crazy, but if you can explain what you're doing, this will save you from the finger prick method and from buying all those test strips. Keep in mind that your insurance isn't going to pay for this since you're probably not diabetic. Last time I looked, they cost about two hundred dollars. If you live in a state that I am licensed to practice medicine in, I'd be glad to help you find access to one. Drop me an email at my contact information in the back of this book.

If you're unable to convince your doctor to prescribe you a glucose monitor, or if you can't afford one, you can still improve your metabolic health. Go to any pharmacy and pick up a glucose meter and testing strips, and follow the instructions to test twice daily. If that's not possible for you, either, then continue the other aspects of improving your metabolic health without the glucose monitoring.

MANAGING WHAT YOU'VE MEASURED

By this point, you've learned everything you need to know about the five markers. Now that you know how to measure, it's time to learn how to manage. Let's talk about what you can do, starting right now, to improve your metabolic health for good, for life.

PART II

PRINCIPLES OF
METABOLIC HEALTH

THE SEVEN PRINCIPLES OF
METABOLIC HEALTH

Now that you know how to measure your metabolic health, it's time to manage it.

Every person reading this book comes from a unique background. Your starting point is specific to your life. That said, since you're reading this book, it's likely you have struggled with some aspect of your metabolic health. Many readers may have decent metabolic health and are looking for skills to maintain it. But with 88 percent of Americans failing at least one metabolic health criteria, odds are your health has potential for improvement.

Beyond the measurements included in the previous chapter, be aware that metabolic health affects your medical health in a variety of ways. Autoimmune disorders like psoriasis and inflammatory bowel diseases are a few serious conditions that often result from a high-carb, processed-food diet. If you're dealing with a severe condition that can be traced back to metabolic health, strict adherence to the following guidelines may help reduce your symptoms.

One of the most common autoimmune diseases I see associated with poor metabolic health is rheumatoid arthritis, which is treated as an unsolvable condition with expensive medication to keep patients functional.[35] If you can reduce or even cure your condition and get your life back without expensive medications, isn't that worth the effort to change?

Use the measurements from the last chapter, including your blood work results and all applicable tests from your doctor, to determine how closely you need to follow the seven principles at the start. (In other words, don't continue reading this chapter until you have your metabolic results).

Once you know how your health currently stands, be realistic. If you're failing five out of five health measurements, you likely need drastic action to pull you out of danger. That means you may wish to follow these standards seven days a week without varying until you've got your health back under control. Someone who passes all five criteria and just wants to lose five or ten extra pounds may not need to be as strict. Then again, they may want to preserve their health. Following this system every single day will keep you healthy, wherever your starting point may be.

As you tailor your experience with the following guidelines, keep in mind this is a lifelong change, not a sprint to health. If self-discipline is a challenge right now, you can always begin slowly and ramp up your strictness as you wean your body off substances like sugar. If you currently follow the typical American diet, every day that you follow these guidelines will improve your health. Those effects can build on each other to make it easier to maintain control of your diet later once you see the initial benefits.

INTRODUCING THE SEVEN PRINCIPLES

If you're going to improve your health, you need a system. The seven principles are a framework for metabolic health designed to get you healthy and keep you there for life.

Why seven principles? Why not nine, or five, or an even ten? Sure, everyone has their program and their arbitrary numbers. But these seven principles are drawn from my experience, both personal and professional. As

---

35 Manole Cojocaru, Inimioara Mihaela Cojocaru, Isabela Silosi, and Camelia Doina Vrabie, "Metabolic Syndrome in Rheumatoid Arthritis," *Maedica* (Bucur) 7, no. 2 (2012): 148-152.

a practicing heart surgeon, I know how to break systems down into working parts. And as I recovered my own metabolic health, I took notes on general topics and themes that kept emerging. These seven principles come up again and again as one learns about and works to improve metabolic health.

Now, you might be asking, "Is this system peer-reviewed? Has it been studied at the Mayo Clinic?" The truth is, no, this is not a peer-reviewed study or a textbook. But as we've established, what those studies and textbooks say is questionable because the established medical system doesn't work, given the 88 percent of people who are metabolically unhealthy. The current system is designed to keep you overweight and on several medications as the sugar industry keeps shoving poison down your throat, and many peer-reviewed journals walk in lockstep with that goal. If you want to get better, you'll need to develop better criteria for figuring out what works instead of trusting compromised experts.

These seven principles are built to help any person at any starting place in their medical health. But it's impossible to give a specific recommendation or even a prescription that's going to work for everyone. If you're looking at your blood work panels and other metabolic health signs, and you're surprised or concerned about the results, yes, these seven principles will help.

However, most people benefit from one-on-one care from a qualified medical professional who is familiar with metabolic health. It's unfortunate that many physicians aren't familiar with or dismiss metabolic health, often because it clashes with the established compromised narrative. When you select a professional to help you, make sure they buy fully into this new system so you aren't fighting an uphill battle with a medical professional who doesn't believe in what you're trying to do.

Since you're reading this book, you recognize that I have expertise in this area. You don't have to work with me personally, but if you like the message of this book, you may enjoy a consultation with my practice, Ovadia Heart Health. If you are so inclined, visit **ovadiahearthealth.com**.

Now that we've introduced the framework, let's discuss each of the principles.

PRINCIPLE 1: REFRAME HEALTH AS A SYSTEM, NOT A GOAL

If you want to get metabolically healthy, the very first step is to get out of the diet and weight-loss mindset.

When most people decide to get healthy, they set arbitrary goals they think sound good. "My goal is to lose this many inches from my waist." It's easy to look at your blood tests and measurements and come up with specific improvement goals. But we've established that a person can be thin and still in metabolic danger, but even setting that aside, there are two key reasons this goal mindset doesn't work.

The first issue with aiming for a specific goal is, once people lose the inches, they go right back to pre-diet eating. "I lost my twenty pounds! Now I can enjoy ice cream cakes again." They load up on sugar, which begins their addiction cycle all over again. This gets worse as something else in their life stresses them out and causes them to increase their sugar consumption to feel better. Then they're horrified to discover they've gained back their twenty pounds plus interest. I know, because this was my own dieting pattern prior to discovering the truth about metabolic health.

The second problem is that most people never reach their original goal. Dieting and weight loss can be hard, and we can plateau even while working hard to get better. Failing to cut out the problem foods will inevitably cap your ability to succeed. And when people don't reach their goal, they give up. The arbitrary goal itself becomes a discouragement.

Think about every major weight-loss and dieting company in the past thirty years. Systems like Weight Watchers earn so much money because they have so many repeat customers. You get on their system and eat better for a while, then switch off their system and gain it back. Then you remember their plan worked, so you pay them again. Rinse and repeat. It's a subscription model that keeps customers coming back for more help.

Even without a system, most diet books are focused on a skill set instead of a mindset. They teach you tips and techniques to make it easier to stick to their diet, but they don't teach you how to change your entire perception so that being healthy becomes second nature rather than a constant battle.

Mindset has to come first. Yes, I'm going to give you practical tips on how to do this, but mindset must come first. You need to know the purpose of why you want to improve metabolic health. Your defining reason will shift your perception from, "Ugh, I have to eat healthy again," to, "I'm going to live a longer and better life because of this meal I'm about to eat."

The best systems, as *Dilbert* creator and *New York Times* best-selling author Scott Adams would say, are ones that you can follow over and over and over almost without thinking about it. Instead of many goals to chase all at once, you need *one* sustainable system you can stick to that improves your health every day. Without thinking twice.

I faced this system-versus-goal mindset in my own weight struggle. I had tried over and over to lose forty pounds, and I dropped some, but I always gained it back. But when I decided to focus on becoming healthy and maintaining my metabolic health, I sucked the energy out of my negative perception of weight. I stopped weighing myself every day and instead focused on how my overall health was changing.

Recently, I saw people on Twitter discussing the pros and cons of intermittent fasting (IF). IF is goal orientation, not systems thinking. "Fast sixteen hours in a row, every day." That's focused on the wrong goal. IF is difficult to the point of unsustainability for many who try because they're hungry all the time. It's either uncomfortable, or they binge during that eight-hour window and eat more calories than they would have without the IF goal. I replied to the Twitter discussion and said, "Eat in such a way that you are hungry less often, which naturally results in a transition to a sixteen-hour fasting window without thinking about it." Just that one shift shocked many people in the discussion, but it led to a deeper conversation about sustainability and systems versus pointless goal setting.

A useful tool for enacting the systems-over-goals principle is called an OODA loop, which stands for **Observe**, **Orient**, **Decide**, and **Act**. The blood panels you should have just received cover observation. Orientation involves a new direction, often by noticing what metabolically healthy people are doing to achieve the results you desire. Reading this book is one way to orient yourself. Then decisions, obviously, mean choices. Another tip I can credit to Scott Adams is deciding versus trying. *Trying* to improve your eating is a single-ingredient recipe for failure. *Decide* you'll do what it takes to improve. Once you've decided, take swift, decisive, consistent action.

The OODA loop has served me well in my metabolic health practice and client coaching. It's a useful framework to actively manage permanent behavioral change and create desired outcomes. And that's exactly what we want for your health.

In Part III, we're going to apply the metabolic health mindset, this principle, to specific diet recommendations. Once you learn to follow systems instead of goals, tackling medical and metabolic health becomes far less intimidating.

PRINCIPLE 2: EAT REAL WHOLE FOOD

You might ask, "What is real whole food?" The answer is simple: real whole food comes from the earth, or it eats things that come from the earth.

Most of your food should not have an ingredients list or label because the food itself is the only ingredient. Food like a banana, a head of lettuce, or a cut of beef. Real whole food is that which you could, theoretically, in the right weather conditions with enough space, grow or raise in your backyard. If it wasn't something your great-grandparents were eating one hundred years ago, it's not something we should be eating now.

How bad is the modern diet? Seven out of eleven of the top causes of death in 2020 were related to metabolic health, including heart disease, cancer, stroke, and diabetes.[36] Even COVID-19, number three on that list, is more harmful and deadly to people with poor metabolic health.

Let's put the statistics into their historical context. Experts claim that we're living longer now, but we really haven't improved our *net* lifespan. That's because, from a statistical standpoint, the experts use reported averages. But a 50 percent infant mortality rate lowers that number significantly. Kids dying in early childhood from preventable issues reduces the net lifespan further. Removing those factors paints a much clearer picture of how long our ancestors lived a hundred years ago, or even a thousand years ago.

Remember that the germ theory of disease was discovered in the 1600s. Over the last three centuries we've increased its application, from handwashing to sewer systems to antibiotics. That helps with preventable diseases like influenza and pneumonia, which in 2020 was the ninth leading cause of death. But we have not improved our health, and in fact we've worsened it because of the food we're eating.

Consider the health of a seventy-year-old today versus a seventy-year-old one hundred years ago. Most people spend the last ten or even twenty years miserably unhealthy these days, stuck in electric wheelchairs or dumped into nursing homes. But even just a few decades ago, people lived healthy until the day they died. Great-grandpa could be eighty years old and still working in the field with the whole family, get the flu, and pass away in forty-eight hours. And he'd have full use of his body his entire life up until his last few hours.

If our infant and child mortality rates are improving, and our handwashing and sanitation has helped, why don't we see massive lifespan increases based on the weighted numbers? Because our food is

---

36 Niall McCarthy, "Covid-19 Was the Third Leading Cause of Death in the U.S. in 2020 [Infographic]," Forbes, last updated April 21, 2021, https://www.forbes.com/sites/niallmccarthy/2021/04/01/covid-19-was-the-third-leading-cause-of-death-in-the-us-in-2020-infographic/?sh=1eab557a5af1.

now poisonous. It's killing us, it takes a long time to die, and we suffer the entire time. Our food robs us of decades of living while we're still alive.

That's why it's crucial to return to real whole food. We also need to address the American food culture and its role in our daily lives. Eating real whole food means eating for nutrition—fueling your body to live your life—not eating as a hobby, social event, boredom cure, or "treat." Your body needs nutrition, not calories. Meet your body's nutritional needs, and you won't need to eat as much.

The truth is that your body tells you when you're full. You don't look for snacks because you're eating nutritionally dense foods. You're satisfied. This is the big difference between larger volumes of nutrient-poor, calorie-dense foods. It's also the difference between not being hungry versus being satisfied. Compare the high-carb Chinese food cooked in vegetable oil. Everyone is hungry an hour after eating Asian versus dining at the steakhouse where everyone is full the rest of the day. They need only a light breakfast the next morning, if one at all.

When you're constantly eating sugar and processed carbohydrates combined with seed and vegetable oils you could be hijacking your body's signals telling you when to eat. Instead of craving nutrients, you might be craving your next dopamine fix or trying to raise your blood sugar after a crash. Eating real whole food stops this endless sabotage and helps you get in touch with your body's natural signals again so you know what you actually need, not what your addicted brain craves.

Finally, real whole food can encompass even extreme diets like carnivore and vegan. Because while they're restrictive, they're usually based on awareness of what exactly is in your food. For most people, the best balance is somewhere in between carnivore and vegan. Because as long as you're not eating processed carbs and vegetable and seed oils, you'll probably be well.

This is the second time I've called out these industrial oils specifically, so I ought to explain why. Vegetable and seed oils are high in omega-6 fatty acids, which are detrimental to the body when consumed in high amounts. The typical high-carb, low-fat diet most Westerners partake of is ironically high in omega-6 fatty acids. And the results have been nonoptimal, to say the least:

> PUFA are increases in chronic inflammatory diseases such as nonalcoholic fatty liver disease (NAFLD), cardiovascular disease, obesity, inflammatory bowel disease (IBD), rheumatoid arthritis, and Alzheimer's disease (AD).[37]

Should you track your intake of omega-6 fatty acids? I don't recommend you do. That's a goal, not a system. Instead, follow our new system—eat real whole food. Industrial oils are not that.

IS THIS KETO? PALEO? LOW-CARB?

This is a fair question. Most dieting books will try to give you a specific name for the eating plan so you can follow an established diet. And switching away from carbs and sugars sounds awfully close to some specific eating plans out there.

But I'm not a big fan of labels because they paint people into a corner. My target for you is not to get you to stick to just one rigid dietary practice, but to make the switch from fake food to real food. If that means your diet starts to resemble keto or paleo, then so be it.

As for me, I don't follow any specific diet 100 percent. For one thing, I don't want to be in the scenario where I'm telling everyone to eat carnivore but get a picture taken of me eating a bagel! Instead, I eat real whole food and keep my metabolic health system in mind. There is no one right way to do this. Remember, you're building a system, not focusing on a goal. I never say, "I never eat that food," I just generally choose to avoid it.

---

37 E. Patterson, R. Wall, G. F. Fitzgerald, R. P. Ross, C. Stanton, "Health Implications of High Dietary Omega-6 Polyunsaturated Fatty Acids," *Journal of Nutrition and Metabolism* 2012 (2012). https://doi.org/10.1155/2012/539426.

And there's a mental benefit to this approach. Almost everyone loves to eat ice cream. So when they start a diet, what's the one cheat food they can't stop thinking about? Ice cream! They fight it for weeks until they have a bad day and give in, and then they feel like they failed. That can spell the end of their dieting attempt. That's why, even with my metabolic health in mind, I still eat ice cream on occasion. But if I eat ice cream, I eat ice cream that is made from simple ingredients like milk, sugar, and vanilla, and I often fast the next morning. That removes the pursuit of perfection and makes this system sustainable. After all, who wants to live a life with no ice cream?

I'm not asking you to give up everything you love for the rest of your life. You need to get your metabolic health under control, and then you can decide for yourself what to reintroduce, how often, and how to balance it against your healthy system.

PRINCIPLE 3: MAKE ONE SUSTAINABLE CHANGE AT A TIME

In *The ONE Thing*, Gary Keller wrote a line that has stuck with me. "What's the one thing you can do such that by doing it everything else will be easier or unnecessary?" That principle is key to understanding metabolic health. By improving this aspect of your health, you improve *all* aspects of your life.

But breaking down metabolic health even further, we can apply this same principle over and over. Changing your entire life can be overwhelming. But changing one thing is manageable. So if you're going to change just one thing at a time, you need to find the best change that will give you the most benefit and make future changes even easier.

If you need to overhaul your medical health but aren't sure where to start, you can look for places where you'll get the most impact first. By looking for the biggest bang for your buck, you simplify your health journey while also gaining motivation from each change you make.

You may have gotten your test results back and felt a little overwhelmed by what seems like a monumental task: uncoupling from the current food and medical system and building a lifestyle that won't destroy you. If you're feeling stressed over the enormity of your task, rest assured that you do not need to make every single change right now. You don't have to wake up tomorrow and eat like you're preparing for the Ironman competition. It's OK not to be perfect right at the start.

Instead, you need to find one key change you can make right now that you can sustain long enough for it to make a difference. Ideally, you'll want to continue that change at least until your medical health improves, and then you switch to following it *most* of the time as you maintain your metabolic health. With that in mind, sustainability is absolutely key.

Here are four suggested changes that will help you eat the metabolically healthy way.

Prioritize. Eat the real whole food first. Most people gravitate to the sugars and carbs first because they feel good to eat. That means they ignore the fancy steak in favor of eating bread and loaded baked potatoes. One easy change is to alter the order you eat your food so that you eat real whole food first. If you've got a plate of food in front of you, eat the steak first, then see if you're still hungry for the white-bread roll. You may just fill up too much to eat many carbs or sugars, which makes resisting them a snap.

Replace. Change out the processed food you typically eat with the real whole food alternative. This may sound complicated but can be simple. It could mean swapping your fried chicken from a frozen bag to real chicken breast from the refrigerated section. Or switching from canned vegetables preserved in oil to the real vegetables from the produce section. Does this require a little extra work? Yes. But if it means the last ten to twenty years of your life are spent running around having fun instead of strapped to an electric wheelchair, isn't that worth spending those extra few minutes cooking?

Substitute oils. Instead of cooking with fake oils—the highly processed and unstable industrial oils like canola oil, sunflower oil, and safflower oil—use real whole foods. Animal fats you can substitute are butter, lard, and tallow. You can find lard and tallow in the baking aisle or the refrigerated section. That's what our grandparents and ancestors cooked with. Fruit fats are acceptable as well. These include coconut oil, avocado oil, and olive oil.

One word of caution for olive oil: up to 80 percent of olive oils sold in the United States contain industrial oils.[38] If it's cheaper than it should be, it's cut with seed oils. Real coconut oil is solid at room temperature. It's harder to corrupt. We're told to avoid meat and animal products because they are high in saturated fat, yet coconut oil, which contains an even higher percentage of saturated fat, is widely recognized as being beneficial to our health. This inconsistent messaging shows how little the healthcare industry actually understands what's in our food.

Replacing these bad oils with good ones also short-circuits a major challenge many patients experience. The typical doctor's diet strategy is to eliminate oils, and your willpower fails because you miss them. That's why I educate people about why those oils are so damaging and teach an overall healthy system with proper balance. The natural thought becomes, "If I want to be healthy, I'll give those specific oils up in favor of healthy ones."

The last suggestion is to **eat fewer snacks**. Real whole foods at mealtime are more nutritionally dense and therefore deliver more of the vital nutrients that we need for less calories compared to processed, packaged food-like products. This is the principle behind high-carb takeout food that leaves you hungry again in one hour. Your body didn't get what it needed, so even if it's not truly hungry, it sends hunger signals to make you snack to get the rest of your nutrients. When you load up on the proper nutrients at meals, you won't need to snack as often, which means fewer calories. That in turn can help you shed weight and not face so many food temptations during the day.

---

38 "Don't Fall Victim to Olive Oil Fraud," CBS News, last updated January 3, 2016, https://www.cbsnews.com/news/60-minutes-overtime-how-to-buy-olive-oil/.

There are other changes to make, but these four sustainable changes, made one change at a time, work wonders for most people. If you're stuck for where to begin, any of these is a great starting point for the road to good metabolic health.

PRINCIPLE 4: MOVE

It's time to get more active throughout your day.

Relax—the goal isn't to have your training for a marathon. Remember, these changes are supposed to be sustainable and easily managed in the course of a normal day. But the truth is that our modern lives have become more sedentary than is healthy for us. We intake calories because our bodies expect to use them. If we don't use them, we just sit, and when we sit we get bored, so we snack. That increases our calorie intake, still without adding any meaningful caloric burn.

To incorporate more movement, focus less on exercise but be more active whenever possible. Just get up and move around. Here are a number of suggestions for easy inclusion in our daily life:

- Use a standing desk or treadmill desk.
- Take the stairs instead of the elevator.
- Park farther away from the store in the lot or on the street.
- Play with your kids and pets actively.
- Take walks with your partner in the morning or evening.
- Do short exercise stints during the credits of each episode you binge of your favorite show or podcast.

These are easy practices anyone can include without disrupting their current lifestyle. And by including all of these into your overall day it will keep you healthier than working out for an hour at the gym while being sedentary throughout the rest of the day. You spend more energy if you are active throughout the day rather than sitting around for fifteen hours with one hour at the gym and another eight hours sleeping.

▨ EXERCISE FOR LIFE

By incorporating constant movement, you build and maintain muscle as you age. It may be challenging to work out at the gym an hour every day in your sixties, but even a person in their nineties can incorporate constant movement. If you really want to build muscle, focus on metabolically healthy exercise. No, that's not cardio. It's lifting and resistance body-weight exercises. And building and maintaining muscle as you age should be the primary focus, because it directly correlates to quality of life.

Consider what's going to impact your quality of life in later years. The Frailty Index measures an elderly person's likelihood of managing daily tasks and surviving accidents.[39] And you want yours as low as possible. Why? Avoiding accidents in particular is associated with strong grip strength, i.e., low frailty. You want to be able to get out of bed, hold on to rails, and walk upstairs without falling when you're ninety, right? There's no reason you have to be confined to a wheelchair or so thin that a strong breeze could knock you over and break your hip. Grip strength alone is proven by research to improve survival rates, help avoid falls, and provide better health outcomes.[40,41]

And if you do fall down in your old age, would you rather be frail and break a bone or loaded with muscle to absorb the fall? And would you rather be too weak to push yourself up or so muscular that you can roll into the push-up position and knock out a few while you're down there? There are people in their nineties right now who can do more push-ups than some men in their thirties.

---

39 Xia Li, Alexander Ploner, Ida K. Karlsson, Xingrong Liu, Patrik K. E. Magnusson, Nancy L. Pedersen, Sara Hägg, and Juulia Jylhävä, "The Frailty Index Is a Predictor of Cause-Specific Mortality Independent of Familial Effects from Midlife Onwards: A Large Cohort Study," *BMC Medicine* 17, no. 94 (2019). https://doi.org/10.1186/s12916-019-1331-8.

40 Richard W. Bohannon, "Grip Strength: An Indispensable Biomarker for Older Adults," *Clinical Interventions in Aging* 14 (2019): 1681-1691. https://doi.org/10.2147/CIA.S194543.

41 Christina Musalek and Sylvia Kirchengast, "Grip Strength as an Indicator of Health-Related Quality of Life in Old Age—A Pilot Study," *International Journal of Environmental Research and Public Health* 14, no. 12 (2017): 1447. https://doi.org/10.3390/ijerph14121447.

▪ INTENSE EXERCISES THAT WORK

You don't need to be a bodybuilder to achieve good results over the course of your lifetime, you just need to maintain a reasonable amount of mass. That means keeping yourself from being overweight but also from being underweight or undermuscled. You can achieve a good balance with easy bodyweight resistance exercises like pull-ups and squats. These can be done in the home with minimal equipment. You can also incorporate any sort of resistance using weights or TheraBands to build and maintain muscle.

If you're willing to get a little more into your personal fitness, invest in a nice set of kettlebells and use them while you watch your favorite shows. Lifting and moving with kettlebells adds extra stress to your frame that boost muscle growth, and you can mimic many normal movements you'll use throughout the day anyway. That way, as you age, your body is used to doing those daily tasks with additional weight. Doing them with your normal weight will seem easier and will keep you safer.

A lot of clients ask me about my personal routine. I use the X3 Bar, so called because you work out to triple failure. It's a series of eight exercises that incorporate a mix of pushing and pulling, with one set of each. You get to a point where you have completely exhausted all the muscles. Doing all eight exercises takes about twenty minutes, and I do that three times a week. John Jaquish writes about the X3 Bar and has called weightlifting a waste of time. For more on that exercise routine, check out his book *Weight Lifting Is a Waste of Time.*

The point is that you don't need to obliterate your body with three-hour workouts every day, like most people imagine is required. For any type of resistance, one set to failure is the biggest stimulator of muscle growth as opposed to many sets and many reps. Do fewer reps with heavier weight. As we discussed before, simply standing and walking around is a form of resistance exercise, and that maintains muscle mass.

■ THE CARDIO CONUNDRUM

If you want to add cardio to your fitness routine, whatever you enjoy is fine. Biking, hiking, running, and rowing are all fine examples. But keep in mind that research shows cardio is an unreliable tactic for fat loss.[42] That's a shock to most people because we've been taught that cardio is *everything*. Jogging was practically the number one exercise in America for a while.

Some cardio can be good for you, even if it doesn't help with weight loss or metabolic health. But you don't need to do anywhere near as much as people imagine. All-out sprinting for twenty seconds, five times, over a ten-minute period, twice a week is more effective than jogging slowly for two hours. Concentrated bursts of intense workout results in significant visceral fat reduction over a week, a month, a year. Sean O'Mara, MD, out of Minnesota, performs MRIs to measure that visceral fat reduction. His work is fascinating, and I recommend you read up on his studies at **drseanomara.com** if you're interested in effective cardio.

If you do incorporate cardio into your life, be smart about it. Running for long distances really just trains you for running long distances. How often do you plan to do that in your life versus living a normal life where you need to maintain balance and metabolic health? Marathon runners actually live shorter lifespans than the average population based on available research. Read up on that shocking fact, and you'll realize that your time is likely better spent elsewhere.

There's no need to gear up for a marathon when working out to your favorite TV show in your own living room will give you better lifelong results. Most of us are time restrained anyway, so I would rather you use it wisely. Exercise while you're living your life. And then, once in a while, do one workout set to failure.

As one last point, let's confront the cardio myth. "Skinny people do cardio." That may be backwards. People who are health focused enough

---

42 Damon L. Swift, Neil M. Johannsen, Carl J. Lavie, Conrad P. Earnest, and Timothy S. Church, "The Role of Exercise and Physical Activity in Weight Loss and Maintenance," *Progress in Cardiovascular Diseases* 56, no. 4 (2014): 441-447. https://doi.org/10.1016/j.pcad.2013.09.012.

to do significant cardio are probably also doing several other things right, which together keep them thin. And obviously the people who are thin have been on the treadmill longer! They're conscious of workouts and calories, so they get results. It just looks like cardio is the magic key.

Then an average person starts doing cardio alone and gets few results. And cardio is hard! Your body resists it because it impacts your joints and burns calories fast. It's the least-optimal state for getting healthy. Besides that, you can't out-exercise a bad diet. All those healthy cardio fanatics also eat whole foods and count their calories.

Instead, focus on constant movement. Being active gives you a little more leeway to tolerate what you wouldn't be able to tolerate without any exercise. And it builds a lifetime of safety and good health that will help you enjoy your old age as you beat youngsters in push-up contests.

PRINCIPLE 5: SLEEP ENOUGH

Read that principle again.

It's not, "Sleep *more.*"

Sleep *enough.*

When you read it, what was the first thing that popped into your head? Probably an amount of time, right? Maybe you did a rough calculation about the average time you sleep. Length of sleep can help in some cases, sure. You're not likely to be healthy at two hours of sleep per night. But more important than sleep quantity is sleep quality.

The number thrown around for optimal sleep is eight hours. But the "eight-hour rule" isn't enough because you need deep sleep for rest and recovery, and the amount of deep sleep you can get varies based on a number of factors. If you're constantly woken up by a screaming baby every fifteen minutes, for example, you won't feel rested even if your partner takes care of the baby while you stay in bed for the full eight hours.

And you may even need less than eight hours to reach your optimal level. In my experience, as patients get metabolically healthy, their sleep improves. This happens because they're not destroying their body with bad food, and they lose weight. As a result, they put less stress on their body, so they need less rest and recovery time. You just don't have as much to recover from at the end of a day, and your body recognizes that.

As a personal example, I get less sleep now that I'm metabolically healthy than I used to need when I was overweight. I never got into sleep tracking devices and measurements of sleep, but I never had a problem with my sleep even when I was overweight. Even without previous disruptions to compare against, the amount has decreased noticeably as I've improved my metabolic health.

Metabolic health improvement means you need less sleep, but it also means you don't spend all day feeling tired. No more chugging afternoon coffee to compensate for sluggishness. A lot of people who drink their calories in the second half of the day are consuming sugary caffeine beverages like Mountain Dew just to keep themselves energetic and awake. Those sugars and calories go back into their system and make them even more sick, which increases their run-down feeling. Repeat, repeat, repeat, every single day, until they end up on my operating table. That cycle only stops once you clean up your metabolic health.

The truth is that it's not normal to feel exhausted every day. Feeling tired means metabolically unhelpful choices were made during the day. Those choices leave you unable to be active throughout the day. But getting good sleep supports your whole body in recovering to the max each night and being prepared for a full day of energy.

■ SIMPLE TIPS TO GET QUALITY SLEEP

When clients ask me about improving their sleep, I talk to them about cultivating the right sleep environment and sleep hygiene. These are unfamiliar terms for many people. Sleep environment means your actual area where you sleep, not just the bed but also the room as a whole and even outside your room. Sleep hygiene, on the other hand, relates to your person both inside and out and how you prepare yourself for good sleep.

Most people stare at their phones while they're lying in bed. This is poor sleep hygiene because your screen has blue light, which can stimulate parts of your brain you don't need stimulated before sleep. For this reason, some people wear blue-light-blocking glasses that prevent their phone from messing with their brain chemistry. It sounds goofy, but this can actually help if you struggle to unwind right before bed and quiet your mind.

And while we're on the subject, it's best not to use screens at all an hour before bed. Stick to normal conversation, paperback books, and other activities that don't shove a bright light in your face.

When you do sleep, prepare your sleep environment the best you can. Give yourself an adequately dark room, or invest in a comfortable sleep mask if you've got lighting issues. Don't leave the TV on all night, even if you like it for company, because the noise can snag your unconscious mind and pull you out of deep sleep even if it doesn't wake you all the way up.

And avoid stimulants prior to sleep. This includes nicotine in cigarettes but also all forms of caffeine. You might be surprised what other items in your daily life are stimulants, so do some research on the topic if falling asleep is a struggle for you.

Make sure you avoid alcohol after dinner. Yes, I know, plenty of people unwind with a glass of wine before bed. This is common enough to be a cliché, but it's actually bad for your sleep hygiene. Yes, alcohol can help you fall asleep faster, but it also disrupts the quality of that sleep as your brain chemistry struggles to return to normal. This effect is significant enough that it can account for a lot of bad sleep all on its own, and people will never know it.

Lastly, consider your caffeine intake and schedule. This has different impacts for each person. Some folks will have multiple espressos with their dessert and be able to sleep like a log. Other people can't even drink coffee after lunch or they'll be awake half the night. Be honest with yourself about your caffeine impact and try adjusting your current schedule to see if your sleep improves.

There is no one right diet, and there is no one right amount of sleep or way to sleep. These tips I've mentioned are things to consider, adjust, and experiment with as you find what works for you. We have no scientific data or even anecdotes to say that what works for one will work for another.

Play around with your sleep environment and sleep hygiene until you find what works best for you.

PRINCIPLE 6: RELIEVE STRESS

Chronic stress worsens metabolic health. Stress causes inflammation, which leads to metabolic syndrome.[43,44] Stress also causes hormonal changes that counteract good metabolic health. And chronically elevated levels of the stress hormone cortisol are associated with poor metabolic health.

Sleep, like stress, is a measure of metabolic health. If you want to improve your metabolic health, you need to relieve stress. But reducing your stress also brings a host of other positive features. You'll experience mental clarity and calm. And the less stress you experience, the more stable your blood sugar and energy levels will be.

Now, am I telling you to quit your job and move to a beach in Hawaii? No. You don't need to live a 100 percent stress-free life to have good metabolic health. As with everything else, this is about bringing your existing levels down to healthy levels.

If your existing life stress is off the charts, you may need to take drastic steps to reduce stress, that's true. That may look like getting professional help, adjusting your employment, or getting help with your relationships. There is a wide array of options for people experiencing severe stressors in their life.

---

43 Yun-Zi Liu, Yun-Xia Wang, and Chun-Lei Jiang, "Inflammation: The Common Pathway of Stress-Related Diseases," *Frontiers in Human Neuroscience* 11 (2017): 316. https://doi.org/10.3389/fnhum.2017.00316.
44 Guarner V. Rubio-Ruiz, "Low-Grade Systemic Inflammation Connects Aging, Metabolic Syndrome and Cardiovascular Disease," in *Aging and Health: A Systems Biology Perspective*, eds. A.I. Yashin and S.M. Jazwinski (Basel: Karger, 2015), 99-106. https://doi.org/10.1159/000364934.

▦ PRACTICAL TIPS TO DESTRESS QUICKLY

But let's assume you're at an average level of stress, which for modern people is still high. For many of us, part of the problem is that we don't add helpful elements to our day that will help manage the normal stress we accrue just through living our daily lives.

Mindfulness can be key to reducing your stress. For some, that means meditation. This is a tried-and-true practice dating back to ancient times that most cultures around the globe have harnessed to manage stress and foster improved mindfulness. And that meditation looks different for different people. Some may approach it through yoga meditation, while others may pray with prayer beads, and a third group may simply reflect on the natural world around them.

Some people find stress relief and comfort in religious practice. If that's you, you might consider investigating the deeper mysteries of your faith or engaging with religious leaders in your local community or online.

Philosophy can bring about great stress relief. Stoicism, for example, cultivates a purposeful acceptance of challenges. It's helpful not only in daily living but also to manage and improve medical issues that may arise from poor metabolic health.

Whatever route you take, mindfulness is a generally helpful practice to keep you rooted in the present rather than worrying about the future. That in itself will reduce your stress levels by not borrowing more stress from tomorrow. Being intentional about what you're doing throughout the day and taking the time to think about situations versus reacting quickly helps relieve stress as you make better decisions and improve your quality of life.

And relaxed people make better health decisions overall. That will make it easier to stick to some of these other changes you need to make. In short: being less stressed makes it easier to be metabolically healthy, and getting metabolically healthy makes it easier to be less stressed. You're already getting metabolically healthy with earlier changes, so managing your stress on top of those changes will get the ball rolling from both sides.

PRINCIPLE 7: GET A DOCTOR WHO GETS IT

This seventh principle and the previous six are united by a "meta" principle: the principle of sovereignty. *You* are in charge of your health. Your metabolism. Your diet and fitness. Your life span. And the quality of life you experience for however long yours lasts. That means your health is not the government's responsibility. Not food manufacturers', farmers', or ranchers'. Pharmaceutical companies are not sovereign over your health, either. Not even your own doctor is. In many cases, these organizations and individuals offer "advice" that only worsens your health. And they are not accountable to you, either. They lose nothing if you die younger and with a lower quality of life than you could have in the way you and your loved ones lose. So again, you and only you are in position to improve your health because you and only you are in charge of it.

Does that mean becoming your own doctor? No. If you buy a car, it's your car. That doesn't imply you should become an auto mechanic. That *does* mean you, a responsible owner, will take your vehicle to a reputable repair shop when it's time. Similarly, if you're going to take your metabolic health seriously, you need to work with healthcare practitioners who "get it." If your doctor doesn't recognize the supremacy of metabolic health over all else, they may continue pushing unhelpful suggestions on you or even try to sabotage your efforts out of misguided care.

How strongly can you push back if your doctor looks at you and says, "Everything you're trying is garbage, you just need to take your medication"? Maybe you can resist that the first time, and even the tenth, but eventually, if you get frustrated, will you give in and take the medications instead of doing the work? Even if you don't, that will be an uphill battle to be taken seriously. It's difficult to work with a doctor who's laughing at your efforts.

And I don't just mean picking your personal family doctor. Make sure the specialists you work with respect what you're trying to do. Your health journey will be so much easier if the experts near you offer advice centered around these principles. A doctor or specialist who points out helpful metabolic health principles and keeps you accountable for them with appropriate tests will be invaluable in your personal growth.

Unfortunately, finding these sorts of doctors and specialists can be challenging. There's not any one specialty or type of medicine that guarantees everyone there will understand metabolic health. Although all physicians deal with the consequences of poor metabolic health, few understand it, because we're taught wrong information based on a compromised medical system controlled by the Big Food industry. Even those who understand a few of the concepts might not be truly onboard with the full practice. Just because someone recommends you take vitamin C and turmeric for inflammation doesn't mean they understand how to reverse the inflammation permanently through diet.

The good news is that many medical practitioners are waking up to the reality that patients aren't getting better. Doctors who understand metabolic health come from all backgrounds and practice areas, from family doctors and heart surgeons to naturopaths and functional physicians who use supplements instead of prescription drugs. And more of them are becoming better educated every day.

SO WHERE DO YOU FIND SUCH A DOCTOR?

By building networks rather than trusting institutions and their advertisements. The sad truth is that helping people avoid serious health conditions does not pay like treating the consequences of poor metabolic health. So major institutions are going to gear their profit machines toward managing the symptoms rather than delivering the cure. This includes major hospitals, large healthcare organizations, partnerships with pharmaceutical companies, and well-known public figures who are supported by a major organization and the drug companies indirectly or directly.

Increasingly, doctors who emphasize and understand metabolic health are separating themselves from the traditional healthcare system. Part of this is because their education places them at odds with institutional colleagues who still believe the incorrect medical model.

To find doctors with whom you can trust your metabolic health, you'll need to mindfully, intentionally work to find them. Many people put less thought into choosing a doctor than finding the perfect pair of shoes. If you just go to the doctor your insurance covers or one near you, you will likely end up with a doctor who follows the orthodoxy. You have to ask your physician questions like you're interviewing them, not just blindly follow their suggestions. If they only recommend medicine for high blood pressure, press them to answer why.

The fact you're reading this book means you're already on that journey. You're unlikely to sit quietly in your doctor's office and take the medicines you're told to take without asking questions. That's a great start. If you're not happy with your current healthcare team, find a new one.

I can tell you about a new organization I've recently joined, the Society of Metabolic Health Practitioners. We're growing a database of metabolic health practitioners patients can trust. Find us online at **MetabolicPractitioners.org** to see if we have any practitioners in your area.

You can also utilize low-carb blogs and forums because they've usually done the legwork figuring out which doctors do and don't play nice with alternate dietary guidelines. Once you start looking and you get into the network, all you need to do is ask for recommendations and referrals. Word of mouth is key, and there are far more non-doctors out there awake about metabolic health than there are doctors, unfortunately. Let your fellow pilgrims on the metabolic health journey direct you to doctors you can trust.

You can also reach out to me at **ovadiahearthealth.com** even if you don't live in Tennessee or Florida where I currently practice cardiac surgery. Via telemedicine, I work with clients throughout the United States. Coaching services are available internationally. And if for some reason we're unable to connect, notice who I follow and interact with on Twitter—my handle is **@ifixhearts**. That's a great way to lead yourself to the right people.

In the meantime, let's apply the seven metabolic health principles to real life, starting with your shopping list.

PART III

HOW TO EAT METABOLICALLY HEALTHY

TIPS, TRICKS, AND TACTICS TO EAT METABOLICALLY HEALTHY

J*ust tell me what to eat, when, and how much.*

That's how I thought once upon a time. Try as I might to lose stubborn fat and get my numbers where they needed to be, I could not get the diet fads to work long term. I bought the books, joined the groups, and posted my progress to stay accountable. Nothing clicked for me until I learned the truth about metabolic health. Get it right, and everything else goes right.

The opposite is likewise true. I learned the hard way that popular diet menus and regimens don't work. They're not made to. And we've established why already—a business needs customers. Customers who meet their metabolic health goals and maintain them aren't exactly a moneymaker.

Still, I feel tempted to offer you an "eat this, don't eat that" list. That seems like it would be helpful. But because there is no *one right way* to eat metabolically healthy, I can't. That would defeat the purpose of the systems-over-goals principle.

Instead, I'm going to offer you general recommendations for your plan that you can personalize as you wish. The simple tips, tricks, and tactics coming your way in this chapter will improve your diet immediately. Then, in the next chapter, I'll show you how to alter popular diets—one of which you may already be loving, like keto or carnivore—to bring your eating as close to the metabolic ideal as possible.

For this chapter, I will suggest meal adjustments and offer snack ideas. I've tried these myself, and they work so well for me and my clients that we don't have to think about them anymore. It's so easy, it's second nature. Because all we're really doing is following the golden rule of metabolic health: **Eat real whole food.** This principle drives every diet decision I make.

So what does that priority look like in everyday life after the initial motivation burst fades? What about from situation to situation? Cooking at home can be simple, but what about eating out? What about those dreaded birthday parties? Let's bring metabolic health into the real world with this practical advice.

SHOPPING LIST HACKS AND RECIPE ALTERNATIVES

The human body requires a range of vitamins, nutrients, and minerals to stay healthy. If you keep eating what you have been, just making alternatives and switches, you may not get everything you need. You want to be eating as much real whole food as possible. That gives you a much wider range of nutrition.

Many food cravings actually don't come from hunger but from some nutritional deficiency. When you eat real whole food, you don't need a bunch of other things because you're getting all your needs met on one plate. Contrast that to when you get a craving and eat a high-carb food. You're hungry again in an hour, right? Because you haven't provided your body with any real nutrition, you just dumped in a bunch of calories.

To figure out if you're eating real whole food or not, read the ingredients list on every packaged food. It's preferable that what you eat doesn't need an ingredients list. Some combinations of foods are still good for you. Not everything in a package is evil poison—just the packages that *also* contain the harmful substances.

Do your reading and make sure your ingredient list only contains normal foods. And keep an eye out for vague keywords like "seasonings" or "natural flavors." Even seasonings have sugars and chemicals or preservatives that are unnecessary. If the description leads you scratching your head wondering what it means, ditch that food. Read different brands and check the labels until you find what you're looking for.

There are some foods that you're going to need to replace completely. A lot of heavy creamers for your coffee have preservative agents or high-fructose corn syrup. But you can find brands that are heavy cream only. You can even just buy heavy cream directly from farmers and use that. Or learn to enjoy your coffee black for the sake of your health. You've got some wiggle room, and there's no one policing your decisions. Just make sure you're selecting foods that are in line with your metabolic goals.

As for me, I occasionally combine heavy cream, vanilla extract, black coffee, cinnamon, and ice in a blender. It's a great low-carb, metabolically healthy Frappuccino substitute. You might be reading this right now and thinking, *That sounds great*—that's the point. You can eat well and still care for your metabolic health. It's all about eating with intention and selecting for nutrition instead of ease or sugar addiction.

One general rule I follow is this: if you've seen an advertisement for it, it's probably high carb. Pasta sauce, for example, just needs to be tomatoes, olive oil, and basil. But many popular brands that have advertising dollars behind them have industrial oils and high-fructose corn syrup. I'm not saying eliminate pasta sauce altogether, I'm saying find better sources. That might mean making your own sauce, or maybe you find a healthy alternative in a different store than you usually shop at.

This may be a great time to learn to cook for yourself. You can buy spaghetti and pasta sauce with refined white flour pasta and a typical jar of sauce that has high-fructose corn syrup, seed oils, and so on. Or you can make your own pasta sauce with basil, olive oil, salt, and tomatoes with zucchini noodles. It's the same dish essentially, but one is metabolically damaging, and one isn't. Most people would prefer the taste and the experience of the all-natural whole-food version once they've broken their sugar addiction. You'll be surprised how much your taste buds will change and what you find you enjoy once your body is cleaned out.

When you start shopping for real whole foods, you'll probably notice something. Everything you buy is on the outside aisle instead of deep inside the store. The vegetable and produce area, meat counter, seafood area, and dairy and egg center will become your primary sources of ingredients. They're really the easiest places to find real whole food because they're the ingredients you use to make recipes. The food inside the aisles will contain those real foods plus a ton of chemicals to keep them fresh inside their containers. So cut through the preserving process and just get the real food.

You may find yourself eating less often. That's fine. Break away from the typical eating schedule. Let your body's signals be a cue to eat. It will tell you what you need and when. If you find yourself craving a steak at lunchtime, you might need the protein. Give your body what it needs.

One last warning: beware foods that promise good health on the box. Like Keto desserts, the substitute can be worse than the original for bread. Gluten-free does not mean metabolically healthy. Many gluten-free foods don't use wheat but use a lot of highly processed ingredients like vegetable and seed oils, so they may not be any better. They won't cause a flare-up for someone with celiac disease or Crohn's, but they don't support metabolic health. Make sure the switch you're making is to something *better* for you. Don't just swap one poison for another.

Now that we've got some general approaches covered, let's talk about specific food choices you can make to cover various meal types.

BEVERAGES

If you drink alcohol, and if you're afraid I'm going to tell you to drop it, you can relax. You can keep your drinks. But you are going to want to make some changes. The lowest-carb alcohols are tequila, vodka, scotch, and bourbon. If you do mixed drinks, use a zero-carb mixer like club soda. Add mint, lemon, or lime for healthy flavorings. Dry red wines are also low-carb.

See? Healthy living doesn't mean you have to remove everything you enjoy. You just need to change up some of your routines.

When it comes to nonalcoholic drinks from cans and bottles, I'm not the biggest fan of using sugar substitutes. Sugar substitutes can trick the brain into thinking you're eating or drinking actual food. Soda is not an essential food for us. Carbonated water or club soda for the fizzy sensation are better than any diet soda.

If you're tempted to splurge on your favorite drinks, be careful. Sugar doesn't really exist as an available food in nature *on its own*. Our ancestors didn't eat sugar. Yes, fruit *has sugar in it*, but that's a far cry from eating refined sugar. Fruit also has fiber and vitamins and minerals that provide your body with what it *actually* needs.

Soda, on the other hand, is literally pure sugar or sugar substitute without nutrition. Our hunter-gatherer bodies aren't used to that. You're drinking but not getting nutrition, so the body sends the signal to *keep drinking*. Anything you consume that doesn't have vitamins or minerals (even water) will trigger this response in the body. You're eating or drinking empty calories (even no calories), but if the liver has to process it, it will send that "eat nutrients please" signal.

So before you consider having a "cheat" soda, remember that it will make all your following food choices harder for the rest of the day until your body recovers. You're sabotaging yourself in advance, and that one soda may turn into three additional bad choices.

BREAKFASTS

Healthy breakfasts can be very simple. Look to whole food. Fortunately, we have a lot of ancestral whole foods for this first meal of the day.

On the other hand, breakfast has also been aggressively attacked by the food industry. There's usually at least one whole aisle dedicated to sugary toaster pastries and sickeningly sweet cereals. And the cartoon characters on the front are specially designed to attract children and get them hooked on sugar as early as possible. It's predatory.

Get away from processed cereals and oatmeals. You don't need a ton of carbs first thing in the morning. Eat eggs, bacon, and sausage that don't have any added ingredients. Steak and eggs work great as a protein blast to start your day strong.

When do you even eat? If you're not hungry, you don't necessarily need to eat breakfast. "The most important meal of the day" is a marketing slogan, not a statement from scientific literature. If you find yourself not hungry in the morning, don't force yourself. You may discover that you naturally engage in intermittent fasting, as your body only wants lunch and dinner. If that's the case, embrace it.

▪ SNACKS

I'm including a section on snacks because people used to poor metabolic health always imagine they're going to need snacks. That's because they're so used to the carb and sugar binge cycle where they need to constantly fill their bodies with more empty calories.

If you eat real whole foods at mealtime, you'll need to eat less in between meals. Snacking really comes from the food industry. Two to three generations ago, they weren't snacking, because snack foods weren't available. At worst, they'd eat a whole food on the go, with a simple biscuit or some dried meat as a quick lunch while they worked.

But if you find that your body still wants to snack, or if you struggle early in the process as your body adjusts, eat whole real food. I go for cheese, nuts, or blueberries. If I'm feeling a sweet tooth, I mix plain whole fat Greek yogurt with cinnamon and a little honey.

For nuts, get raw or dry-roasted. Most packaged nuts are cooked in vegetable and seed oils. Macadamia nuts, walnuts, and almonds are better to eat than peanuts. If you're going to eat peanut butter or nut butter snacks, just get nuts and salt. Most store-bought peanut butters have vegetable oils and added sugar.

DESSERTS

Just like snacks, if you're eating real whole food, you'll crave desserts less. Desserts should be minimized at most, if not eliminated. Your dinner should be mostly protein so you won't be hungry.

But desserts are baked into our food culture, so you may struggle to get away from them. If so, you can find ice cream and gelato made from simple ingredients, like cream, cane sugar, and vanilla. Compare that to the regular stuff, which is packed with corn syrup solids and vegetable oil. Want to avoid store-bought ice cream altogether? You can also make simple homemade ice cream. You may still be eating some sugar in that sweet homemade goodness, but if you've eliminated it in the rest of your diet you can allow yourself to enjoy some now and then. Who's going to stop you? The only person responsible for your metabolic health is you. Even I enjoy ice cream once in a while.

A word of caution: keto and low-carb ice creams advertised in supermarkets and on social media are really no better than processed ice creams. I would rather you eat a regular ice cream with cream, vanilla, and sugar than overly processed "keto low-carb" ice cream because it's just a marketing gimmick. Sometimes "low-carb" substitutes are worse than what they are trying to substitute for.

For cakes and cookies, look for the cleanest possible. It's hard to find premade cakes and cookies without vegetable and seed oil. That means making them at home. Focus on high-percentage dark chocolate, which usually just includes cocoa and sugar with no extra ingredients.

All of these tips amount to a system-level recommendation: **Prepare your own food, make your own food, cook your own food.** If you're the one preparing all the food from real ingredients, then you know what's in it. You don't have to worry what chemicals the producers might have slipped into that jar.

I've also got options for more restrictive diet choices. Carnivore dieters can blend eggs, stevia, vanilla, whole milk, and butter. Whip it up, put it in the oven, and it forms a cake-like dessert. Cheesecake can be made with eggs, cream cheese, butter, vanilla, gelatin, and stevia.

There are many examples out there to make dessert-like foods healthy from simple ingredients. And because it's real whole food, you don't need to eat the whole package. You can save the rest for later or even make tiny portions so you're not tempted.

■ REAL WHOLE FOOD

You might wonder why you have to cut out 80 percent of the grocery store. Fake food is easily manufactured and overabundant. It's a solution without a problem. That's why it is designed to keep you hungry. Look at potato chips and artisan breads. Do you think we need these things in our diets? Can you picture your ancestor plucking snack chips off a tree?

Don't just eat for the calories. Eat for nutrition and health. That doesn't mean eating has to be miserable or that no meal should be enjoyable. I very much enjoy what I eat. But I know I need to get adequate nutrition and support my health with what I put in my body.

So stick to real whole food. Follow that simple rule, and you'll do great. This gets you away from diet and restriction mentality and allows you to explore new options. Just make sure your choices are actually good for your body.

DEALING WITH RESTAURANTS, EVENTS, AND PARTIES

Everyone who sets out to change their eating habits inevitably dreads going out to eat, celebrating holidays, and attending parties. That's because the biggest temptations pop up around social eating events. This is also where people are encouraged to gorge on sugar and carbs.

You don't have to dread social eating. Remember that I told you that you need a sustainable eating plan, not a restrictive one. Sustainable means you can weather any social eating event without destroying your overall metabolic health. It's all about priorities and choices.

When you eat at a restaurant, make sure you eat the real whole food before you eat processed food and carbs. You may order a steak and get a baked potato with a biscuit and green beans. Eat the steak and green beans first and see how full you feel. Instead of a burger and fries, order two or three burger patties without the bun. If you are still hungry for a side, opt for the baked potato with real butter instead of the fries soaked in vegetable oil.

Following this eating pattern will change the way you think about restaurant eating. You'll find yourself less hungry for appetizers, sides, and dessert. High-carb appetizers like tortilla chips and bread before a meal make you hungry. They're packed with salt, fake fat, and high-carb grain to make your brain crave more food. That's why they're called appetizers.

If you're at a social gathering, find your whole-food options. Meat and cheese trays at events are good. Eat a little at home before you go to the party so you're not starving. You should be able to enjoy yourself without eating or drinking unnecessarily. You can even get more out of the event if you're not focused on eating. But if you show up ravenous, you'll probably gorge on the sugar and carbs first to satisfy your depleted body.

And keep your foods simple. Leave off or scrape off sauces. Many of them are loaded with sugar to make you crave more. Any type of salad dressing is going to have vegetable and seed oils. If you're out and can't verify the dressing's ingredients, go with olive oil and vinegar. These are simple foods and add a little moisture to the food, which is all sauce is really going to do.

If you can guess accurately what ingredients are in it, it's probably real whole food. Stick to the easily identifiable plates. But sauces and sides and casseroles are always going to be an issue because the cook can hide a ton of ingredients inside them. Alfredo sauce is one example that can come loaded with a host of metabolically harmful foods and you'd never know.

You can always just ask and make specific requests. It's not rude to ask the server at a restaurant for a list of ingredients or for your food to be prepared a certain way. For example, ask for your fish to be prepared in butter, not margarine or vegetable oils. You can also just ask for protein without the sides. You can make a combined plate of protein, like steak and shrimp or steak and fish. Order two plain burger patties with cheese, lettuce, tomato, other vegetables without the ketchup (loaded with sugar and chemicals), other condiments, and bun. Don't be afraid to ask for what you want. This is your body on the line here. Don't let anyone stop you from being healthy.

And really, at events and on vacations, you should not need food to enjoy the experience. Focus less on the food and enjoy the experience more. People spend too much time constantly worrying about eating or feeling hungry a lot. Focus on the experience, not the food. You won't look back twenty years from now and remember the food you ate.

And while you *can* eat at restaurants and events, remember to prepare things at home whenever possible. Even if that means you just eat a little ahead of time so you don't arrive starving and make poor choices. And it's OK to decline to eat while you're out. Who can blame you, if you're preparing excellent food at home?

Someone else may be preparing the food, but you have to live with the consequences on your body and in your life when you eat it.

MAKING HEALTHY CHOICES ... MOST OF THE TIME

With any of these tips, you don't have to be perfect 100 percent of the time. Sustainable eating is not about perfection of absolute control. Even *I* don't eat a completely perfect diet—and I wrote a book on metabolic health.

If you do choose to indulge in a food that you normally wouldn't eat, make the intentional effort. This is not a diet you have to be perfect with. It's OK to occasionally enjoy things that don't support your metabolic health. Awareness is really what counts. The next morning, go back to eating a metabolically healthy way.

I want you to remember that this is not all-or-nothing eating. This is about your body, not following my diet. Don't even criticize yourself for indulging. Just be mindful of your metabolic health and know which foods support that long term and which don't. Then make consistent, mindful choices. It's a system, not a goal.

Mindfulness, sovereignty, and personal agency carry the day here. The more you practice and learn, the better you'll get. And the healthier you become, the more you can choose to indulge without dire consequences. Then again, as you become healthier, you'll probably want to indulge less because you feel so good eating clean food.

I tell all clients that the priority is *not* perfection. It's sustainable decision-making. If you're unable to eat a certain way long term because the plan is too complex or the meals too expensive and time consuming, it's better to find another way. My hope is that this chapter's tips will help make metabolic health the natural result of choices that are easier than you expected.

In the next chapter, we'll move from targeted advice to broad plans so you can make eating in a metabolically healthy way part of your existing dietary preferences.

HOW TO EAT METABOLICALLY HEALTHY ON FIVE POPULAR DIETS

I f you're like most people who buy nutrition books, you probably picked up this book hoping for detailed dietary guidelines. After all, that's what most of us are taught to expect. "If you want to lose weight, you need to follow this strict program." Commercials, friends and family, and even doctors tell us this.

You know by now that's not true. Metabolic health doesn't exist solely inside of one diet. Because metabolically healthy eating is a *principle*. Your meal, snack, and beverage choices must align with your metabolism, not some fad.

Are there some eating plans that stick more closely to this principle? Definitely. The Standard American Diet (SAD, an appropriate acronym) is about as far from metabolic health as you can get. Eating 3,000-plus calories per day of fast food, processed snacks, and candy and then sucking down another 2,000 calories in sugary drinks is killing us. It was killing me before I learned everything I've taught you in this book. It was probably killing you, too.

Now you know better, and you want to do better. So you're turning to the one thing most of us understand: a restrictive diet. I can respect that. It's where I started, too. Over time, you'll likely learn to build your own custom diet that works just for you. I've built the Philip Ovadia diet that feeds my body exactly what it needs without filling it with things that might kill me. You'll do the same.

But if you're looking for a place to start, it's best that we examine the top five most popular diet models in America. I'll show you how each one is in line with the guiding principles of good metabolic health. I'll also warn you about the unique challenges each diet will bring to your life. After that we'll discuss a few metabolically healthy meal options you can start with for each diet.

I'll repeat once more that I don't necessarily encourage you to grab one of these diets and stick to it religiously. Instead, if you're looking for a place to start, you can pick and choose some of the options below and build your own diet over time. If you already follow one of these diets, I'll give you new points to consider to make sure you're eating optimally for your needs. The sample meals from each program are all healthy options that will foster good metabolic health. And they're not the expensive, time-consuming recipes that a lot of other books give. These are quick, healthy, inexpensive options to get you started eating better from the moment you close this book and for the rest of your life.

I'm here to help you exercise your agency and take control of your health, whether you decide to go paleo or vegetarian. And you can share this information with others. The eating information you're about to read won't go out of style. What you're about to learn can guide you for the rest of your life. So let's talk about the five most popular diets in America and see how they stack up.

HOW TO EAT METABOLICALLY HEALTHY ON THE CARNIVORE DIET

■ WHAT'S THE CARNIVORE DIET?

The carnivore diet is exactly what it sounds like. You switch to eating purely animals and animal products. That obviously includes meat like beef, pork, poultry, sheep, fish, and game meats, and also foods *from* animals like butter, milk, cheese, eggs, and a wide range of dairy products from animals other than just the cows that most of us might think of.

People are often startled and skeptical the first time they hear about the carnivore diet. "What? You can survive by only eating meat?" The short answer is yes, so long as you're careful and educated. Just like lions and wolves in the wild, human carnivores especially target organ meat like the liver. Liver itself is a true superfood with more concentrations of vitamins and minerals than any other food, even leafy greens and other vegetables, especially folate, iron, and choline, which are essential for your body. And all of those nutrients are already present in bioavailable form so your body digests and uses them easily.

This is actually how most predatory animals in the world get their vitamins, by eating the livers of herbivores who absorb nutrients from plants. The same principle applies to humans. That's why it's necessary to be educated to make this diet work. While some have maintained a long-term carnivore diet without eating organ meats, I recommend them as a good source of the vitamins and nutrients needed to round out a carnivore diet.

MY EXPERIENCE WITH CARNIVORE

I currently have a *mostly* carnivore diet because I find that it's closest to ideal metabolic health for my body's unique needs. But I didn't start out this way.

You probably recall my personal story about being overweight. I struggled my entire life with trying to slim down and get healthy. I tried every fad diet, but nothing seemed to work. And it was hard to stick to extreme restrictions during long work shifts and intense pressure at school.

To shorten the story, I went from the awful SAD eating style to low-carb to carnivore. The longer trail looked like low-carb with gluten-free first, then low-sugar, then keto, then *very* low-carb keto, then carnivore. Low-carb eating was a huge change for me and taught me a lot about how my body processes various foods. I'd been able to lose weight before, but it always came back. When I went low-carb, I lost the weight and finally kept it from coming back. I also saw a host of other positive changes like increased energy and decreased headaches.

The changes were so powerful that I couldn't go back to my old way of eating. I wanted to do even better. I removed sugar next, then reduced my carbs like I was on a crusade against them. I felt better with each additional move. Keto took me up another step. From there I figured, why not make the jump and go all the way?

I went full carnivore in March 2019. I've been *mostly* carnivore for two and a half years now, as of this writing. The biggest change I noticed was reduced inflammation. I had plantar fasciitis and could not get rid of it even with low-carb. It made me miserable for two years. But my third day of carnivore was the first time that my right foot didn't hurt, and it never came back. That pain reduction was enough to sell me on carnivore, but there have been so many other positive changes as bonuses. Whether it was carbs or keto products with seed and vegetable oils in them, there was still something in my diet triggering inflammation. That was eliminated and healed with the carnivore diet.

The other thing I noticed with carnivore was a major boost from the higher protein. I've gained much more muscle mass and maintained it much more effectively, which helps metabolic health. It was like switching muscle growth from hard mode to easy. Although I was lighter on low-carb and keto, I was not as lean, meaning my body fat percentage was higher. Carnivore bulked me up and made me lean as my muscles increased.

Will you see the same results? It's possible. Everyone is different and has different needs. But if you've struggled like I have, you may find yourself enjoying the benefits of the carnivore diet.

▪ PROS OF CARNIVORE

The number one benefit of the carnivore diet is that your nutrients are instantly bioavailable. That means it's the closest to the form your body can use right away, as opposed to undergoing enzymatic changes. Your body needs to break down other foods, and some people because of genetics don't have those enzymes readily available. It's extra work. But when you get your nutrients from animals, whatever animal you're eating has already done that work for you. You're piggybacking off their metabolic work and shortcutting your own process.

The carnivore diet makes a lot of sense when you consider our genetic history. Our ancestors evolved as hunter-gatherers, with hunting making up the majority of our ancestors' diet. It's hard to make the argument that we should change something our species has done for the vast majority of our existence as humans. It's even harder to believe this could be unhealthy. But still, scientists say, "Red meat is unhealthy." How did we all of a sudden start thinking that? We've been eating red meat for 99.99 percent of our species' history.

You read my chapter on nutrition myths. You know how these lies start and who supports them.

Eating meat is not difficult for most people. From a Western religious standpoint, I have yet to find a religion that bans meat (except Seventh Day Adventists, a newer religion). Sure, some religions like Judaism and Islam have rules and rituals and restrictions around what types of meat you can eat, required animal care, and mandatory preparation needs. But these religions enjoy a healthy consumption of meat. Even Eastern religions only have restrictions around meat consumption as opposed to outright bans on meat. For example, many devout Hindus eat poultry and eggs.

If eating meat is a struggle for you, you may need to ask yourself some hard questions. What is your priority? Relying on religion for your metabolic health may be discordant. If your priority is health, that might mean compromising on some of these religious, moral, or ethical principles. From my professional perspective, it's worth it (and I'm also not that religious of a person).

Another major benefit of the carnivore diet is the speed and simplicity of shopping. It gives you a simple shopping list, simple prep, very little cleanup, and an uncomplicated way to eat. We don't need variety and "balance," as those are marketing terms to sell more processed foods. Look at carnivores in the wild or even our pets. They eat the same thing every day for their entire lives. This simplicity is one major reason I've stayed carnivore. It just makes life so easy.

The last benefit is that commercialization or bastardization of this diet is very difficult to pull off. There aren't a bunch of food companies manufacturing cheap products for the diet and blasting you with messages that you *must* eat their products if you want the *full carnivore experience*. If you put refined sugar in jerky or cook pork rinds in soybean oil, it's no longer carnivore. So foods in bags and boxes just aren't going to work for this diet. That protects you from wasting your money.

PITFALLS OF CARNIVORE

I'm going to be as objective as I can, but it may sound like I'm biased. Because the only pitfall of the carnivore diet is realizing you can survive on animal products alone.

Look at the arguments against carnivore. Most people say you won't get variety, or that you'll suffer from the saturated fat content. The fat claim is really a non-argument. See *Fat Fiction*'s top arguments for why it's not an area of concern. As for variety, that's a marketing gimmick from the food industry. You don't really need to be packing your diet with a huge range of foods that your ancestors would never have had access to. Additionally, there is plenty of variety within the carnivore framework. Meats and organs from ruminant and nonruminant animals, seafood, and dairy products can be eaten in many combinations.

Some nutrition groups claim that vitamins and minerals are unavailable in meat. The most common target is vitamin C, a lack of which leads to scurvy. But fresh meat was actually a treatment for scurvy because of the bioavailable content of vitamin C. Sufficient amounts of vitamin C can be acquired from liver or fish roe and eggs. Lower amounts are also present in raw meat and fish. The real issue is that vitamin C is present in *fresh* meat, but not preserved or processed meat. This means you can't just eat fast food burgers and get your required content. And the more carbohydrates you eat, the more vitamin C you need.

You can overcome all of these concerns by eating smart. The carnivore diet really demands that you eat fresh whole food anyway, so you're going to get your required nutrition. All the arguments against this diet are based on the assumption that you'll use a half-baked version in line with the SAD, just focusing on more meat. As long as you do carnivore correctly, don't expect nutrition issues.

HOW TO EAT METABOLICALLY HEALTHY ON KETO, PALEO, ATKINS, OR OTHER LOW-CARB DIETS

WHAT'S A LOW-CARB DIET?

Keto, paleo, and Atkins are members of the low-carb diet family. They diverge based on which carbs they are OK with and which they're not. Here's a handy breakdown of which carb sources each diet plan typically accepts:

Keto

- Avocados
- Tomatoes
- Spinach
- Mushrooms
- Cauliflower

Paleo

- Raspberries
- Strawberries
- Blueberries

- Yeast
- Avocados

Atkins
- Avocados
- Bell peppers
- Cucumbers
- Green beans
- Carrots

General Low-Carb Diet
- Almonds
- Eggs
- Seafood
- Broccoli
- Grapefruit

You might see some overlap, like avocados, but each diet focuses on the low-carb approach in a specific way. Keto tends to stay away even from fruits with high natural sugars and encourage more fats, where paleo says that natural sugary fruits are OK because our ancestors would have picked them off a bush to eat. Atkins encourages a lot more veggie and fiber intake but also allows you to eat special breads branded for the diet. Low-carb is basically a general approach that wants you to stick below a certain amount of daily carbs while encouraging you to eat more meat and fiber instead so you feel full.

The principle they all share is that carbohydrates are dangerous in large amounts, so you need to learn to limit them and replace them with other things. That's the key to remember: *replacement*. These diets assume you're going to crave certain things and need to fill up on others to distract yourself. That's a key difference from the carnivore or vegan diets, which steer you *toward* certain foods, and it's a reason many people can't stick to these low-carb diets. You spend your whole time telling yourself what you're not allowed to eat instead of what you should be looking forward to. That's tough when your willpower dips after a hard day.

PROS OF LOW-CARB

Clearly, limiting carbs is helpful to your metabolic health. These diets all get that right. The evidence is clear that if you take someone who is metabolically unhealthy and limit their carbs, their metabolic health will improve. My own journey began with low-carb because it was an easy change to understand and implement.

The major question is, how low should you go? For some of my clients and patients, I recommend 100 gm. of carbs or fewer. How much of a change is that? The SAD typically includes 300 to 400 gram of carbs per day. Lowering that to 100, or even to 50, is an instant improvement.

Where should you be? If you have high blood sugars or an elevated hemoglobin A1c issue, if your insulin levels are not low, and if all five markers of metabolic syndrome are present, go lower. The lower you go on your carbs, the better.

Do you have to drop to absolute zero? Probably not. The more active you are, the more carbs your body can tolerate. Marathon runners can pack in the carbs and then burn them off. But the SAD level of carbs is built for an Olympic athlete. If you don't have your sights set on a gold medal, odds are good you need to reduce your current levels to improve your health.

For all these reasons, the low-carb diets are an excellent starting place for most people. They won't steer you wrong because you're implementing the initial changes you need to make right now. You can always refine your diet later to a better specific diet that meets your unique needs. And these diets still allow you to enjoy most of the foods you're used to experiencing, so you don't suddenly lose out on everything you've ever loved. That's a huge selling point for these diet models over more extreme changes like carnivore.

▦ PITFALLS OF LOW-CARB

All low-carb diets have been commercialized. They have their own junk food brands and labels. You might think you're eating healthy because the box advertises that the processed food inside meets your dietary requirements, but that doesn't mean it's good for you. You can find junk food with vegetable and seed oils that's "keto" and "paleo," but they are gluten-free processed substitutes. It's not real whole food. It can be tough to sort out which of these foods are actually going to help you meet your metabolic goals.

Because of that, these diets can be deceptive. You may lose weight because you've cut your carb intake but not see improvements to the five signs of metabolic health. That's because your processed foods might be failing to follow the seven principles of metabolic health. Many of these food products still contain these fake fats that the body cannot metabolize properly and are uniquely damaging to the body on a cellular level.

Even worse, Atkins frowns on red meat, and the ketogenic diet focuses on fats over protein. You can load up on unhealthy processed fats and believe you're doing fine, when in fact your body is still struggling. And because you're cutting out natural sources of nutrition your genetics are made to utilize, you're not eating the natural diet your body expects.

HOW TO EAT METABOLICALLY HEALTHY ON THE MEDITERRANEAN DIET

▦ WHAT'S THE MEDITERRANEAN DIET?

The name is actually deceptive, which isn't a good start. This isn't about eating foods that Mediterranean people eat but replicating their lifestyle. That includes lots of walking and sunshine, building a strong community, and engaging with your religious faith. The goal is to develop holistic health in every area of your life. I definitely support this idea. But the diet itself may not work for everyone.

▦ PROS OF MEDITERRANEAN

The absolute best improvement with the Mediterranean diet over the SAD is the strong emphasis on real whole food. They encourage a lot of seafood dishes with fresh vegetables in a light sauce, or baked meat dishes with plentiful fresh herbs. The focus is to eat real food and then take care of your body with light exercise. They also encourage longer meal times so you digest better, and to make eating a fun group activity instead of gorging on fast food alone in front of your television.

This is really more of a lifestyle than a diet, and the lifestyle changes can be particularly helpful for individuals who've closed themselves off from the world and use food to manage their emotional challenges. Learning a better relationship with food is a huge bonus on top of the nutritional changes.

▦ PITFALLS OF MEDITERRANEAN

The Mediterranean diet tends to focus on leaner foods. That means it minimizes meat overall and red meat in particular, which is not the case when you look at Mediterranean countries. They love meat and fat!

This diet also includes lower protein and higher carb intake than is useful for people who are metabolically unhealthy. For example, they'll serve you a lot of pizza and pasta dishes. They're just careful about portion sizes, so you eat less of it. That can leave you feeling hungry, so you might eat twice the amount, at which point you've already blown the diet.

The Mediterranean diet also encourages a lot of olive oil use. That's great if you have access to real olive oil, but most American stores only stock lower-quality olive oil mixed with vegetable and seed oils. This happens because the food labeling guidelines in the United States allow seed and vegetable oils to be in "olive oil" without disclosing that on the label. Food manufacturers include these cheaper oils to increase their profit margin. Our food industry even poisons us when we think we're eating healthy. It's hard to verify that large commercial brands are pure olive oil, not olive and canola (rapeseed) blends. I've heard that "pure olive oil" is allowed to be up to 40 percent *non*-olive oil. That means most store-bought brands are not real olive oil.

The good real stuff gives you a little pinch in the back of your throat. But real olive oil is prone to going rancid quickly. Long shelf life and long expiration dates indicate it's not the real stuff.

If you want to try this diet, here are three olive oils I can personally vouch for as of the time of this writing:

- Selo Olive Oil
- Villa Cappelli
- Kirkland (Costco)

Struggling to find and stock good olive oil is why I prefer lard, butter, and tallow. That can be tough on the Mediterranean diet, which encourages lower fat content and smaller calorie counts.

HOW TO EAT METABOLICALLY HEALTHY ON THE GLUTEN-FREE DIET

WHAT'S A GLUTEN-FREE DIET?

Gluten-free was the very beginning of my metabolic journey. In 2015, before I committed to low-carb eating, I cut out gluten. My perspective changed through the years until I reached full carnivore in 2019.

I felt better as soon as I went gluten-free. It was a huge change, like flipping a switch, and I knew I'd never go back. I had more energy and better mental clarity. I wasn't exhausted every afternoon. And the meager weight loss I'd managed before improved. Then it took off, and I lost a lot more than I'd ever managed on previous diets.

From my experience, there seems to be some autoimmune overlap between celiac diseases and type 1 diabetes. Folks who have one are often at risk for or have markers for the other, even if it's just a gluten sensitivity. Gluten just appears to be bad for us.

Did I have sensitivity to gluten? I didn't know. I still don't, because I never bothered to test it. After experiencing the initial changes, I was hooked. I knew I was never going back to gluten. And I haven't.

PROS OF GLUTEN-FREE

Going gluten-free is often a huge improvement for people. If you have digestive issues in particular, gluten-free diets will help improve GI tract inflammation. This is a major source of irritation, bloating, and metabolic sickness, so this one change could be a key to fixing your health.

And gluten-free is a backdoor way to reach low-carb eating. This is because most processed carbs have gluten in them. Becoming more aware of the gluten content means you're more careful about eating in general, and you're going to gravitate away from a lot of processed foods. When I went gluten-free, I stopped eating bread, pasta, and other products altogether because there weren't that many substitutes. Elimination (not substitution) results in a lower carb intake.

All of those improvements for one simple change is an excellent deal. If you've been on the fence about where to start, gluten-free could be your ticket through the door. Everything else can come after as you see changes take place.

PITFALLS OF GLUTEN-FREE

Gluten-free mass-market products are just as processed if not worse than gluten products. You're trading one problem for another. Gluten-free high-carb products with vegetable and seed oils are not going to be of any benefit to your body. Swapping normal processed food for gluten-free junk means that going "gluten-free" alone won't benefit you as much as you probably need.

This can be a great entry point, but it's really just that. Don't expect your whole life to change, especially if you eat the processed alternatives.

HOW TO EAT METABOLICALLY HEALTHY ON THE VEGETARIAN AND VEGAN DIETS

▓ WHAT ARE THE VEGETARIAN AND VEGAN DIETS?

There are a range of "plant-based" diets based on cutting out meat and other animal products. Some do this for dietary reasons, while others have ethical concerns about the food industry and its treatment of animals.

A rough explanation of the difference is that vegetarians tend to cut out all meat but still eat animal products like cheese, milks, and eggs. Pescatarians typically follow a no-meat diet but include fish plus other animal products like milk, gelatin, and honey. And the vegan diet is entirely devoid of meats and animal products and relies completely on plant-based food sources for nutrition.

Lately there has been a larger push in the media and corporate sectors for plant-based alternatives, especially to beef. The so-called "Impossible Burger" has made its appearance at many fast-food chains. Many wonder at the impact of switching from natural food sources to lab-designed plant-based foods, though the research remains sketchy for now.

▓ PROS OF PLANT-BASED

If a person eats the vegetarian, pescatarian, or vegan diet correctly and educates themselves on their body's nutritional needs, they'll be eating whole foods. The challenge is meeting your entire body's requirements with few or zero animal sources. This diet can seriously deplete a body's nutrients if not handled correctly. But I do know some vegans who sustain this lifestyle long term so long as they supplement in a smart, thorough manner.

I will give veg dieters this, though: The best part of their diet is that it completely eliminates a ton of junk food. Since almost everything in the SAD has animal products, even in foods you may not expect such as Jell-O (gelatin is basically cow bone ashes), vegans cut out the vast majority of fake food that kills so many each year.

▨ PITFALLS OF PLANT-BASED

My top concern with the vegan diet in particular is deceptive marketing. The vegan or plant-based diet is positioned as short-term superior to the SAD, which it is. That's not the problem, though. "Lowers your LDL cholesterol" claims appear often in vegan-supporting studies. Yes, an entirely vegetable diet decreases LDL cholesterol, but lowering it is unclear as a good outcome measure, from my perspective. I don't even see low LDL as a sign of metabolic health. To get better, you need to look at your overall metabolic health, not just lowering your LDL and losing weight.

Now, because vegans are cutting out meat and animal products, you're going to be eating more carbs. Higher-carb diets often mean your triglycerides are high, blood sugar is high, and HDL low. I'd rather people focus on metabolic health overall, not just a few metrics that may improve on the vegan diet but are not outcome related to metabolic health.

The vegan diet may also be labor intensive. Shopping and prepping can be a chore. Exotic ingredients to pull in your full nutritional load may cost a fortune. And your fresh ingredients can go bad much more quickly compared to meats and animal products. Plus, the recipes are complex as you try to replace everything with a plant-based alternative. That means most people won't have the time or money for this extravagant system.

You also need to eat a lot more often. Think of animals in the wild. Carnivores eat once a day; herbivores never stop eating. It's hard to combine fasting with vegan. The vegans I know graze all day. You see that in herbivores in the wild, like chimpanzees. They sit there and eat their entire day, constantly munching on grasses. But with carnivore, I eat one meal a day. If that's what my busy day requires, I don't suffer for it. I get all my nutrition in one blast, and my body retains it all day.

And like I said, low-carb vegan eating is difficult because you've cut out almost everything that *isn't* carbs. When I tried it, I felt lousy because I wasn't low-carb, even though I was vegan. Those carbs left me inflamed and bloated. And because these plant-based diets are so trendy, they're commercialized to death. Marketing just keeps coming up. Processed vegan and vegetarian products are just like keto products—high in seed and vegetable oils. And you're eating a lot of processed grains to try to get full, which have even more of those damaging oils.

Then there's the point-blank fact that supplements are mandatory. Many nutrients do not exist in easy-to-find-and-prepare vegan foods from the grocery store. That's perhaps the biggest trade-off. The long-term successful vegans I know all have a regimented supplement schedule that balances out all the nutrients they're missing, and they're happy that way. Most make this sacrifice for personal or ethical reasons, so they feel positive about supplementation. For vegans, the most significant nutritional supplementations I see are:

- Low-carb / no-carb sugar-free protein sources (organic, clean powders)
- Essential amino acids like creatine
- Vitamin B12
- Adequate iron and folate
- Omega-3 (which you may not need that much of if you're eliminating omega-6 oils)

I suggest vegetarian-adjacent dieters eat eggs and fatty fish like salmon and tuna, both of which are high in omega-3 (that wouldn't work for vegans, but again, it's a trade-off). And I refer vegans and vegetarians to people like Dr. Carrie Diulus, a keto vegan who is also type 1 diabetic, and Dr. Casey Means, who runs a popular vegan Instagram account (@drcaseyskitchen) with metabolically healthy vegan meal ideas.

Done well, the vegan diet has worked wonders for some individuals. As I said, I know several people personally who went vegan and never looked back. But you've got to do it carefully, and you must keep up on your full range of supplements. For people used to eating packaged, processed food, going straight vegan is not easy or cheap to maintain. Several noisy vegan activists announced on social media that they abandoned the diet after the initial switch from SAD to plants. That was probably why. Just because the label features words like "plant-based" and "all natural" does not mean you should eat the food product. It's more of an industrial product than a real food.

This is not to say I do *not* recommend veganism. I do, if done with metabolic health as the priority. Here's why: When I shared an early draft of this manuscript with Dr. Means, she offered a few suggestions. As a long-term plant-based metabolic health advocate, Dr. Means agrees that it is easy to do the vegan diet *very* wrong. Canola oil is vegan; white flour is vegan. That doesn't mean vegans should eat either in large quantities— or at all. That said, Dr. Means told me that doing vegan right can be transformational—assuming a clean, whole food version, as I've mentioned. It's noteworthy that the best metabolic health markers Dr. Means has had in her entire life have been while on a 100 percent vegan diet. In her words, it's been easy to maintain. All she really ate were various combinations of beans, legumes, tofu, vegetables, low-glycemic fruits, nuts, seeds, and spices. No grains, no oil, no refined sugar, no gluten, and just a small amount of starchy vegetables.

In short, veganism can work for you—if you work for it. I've incorporated a few of Casey's meal suggestions in the "Day in a Life" section below.

CONCLUSION: YES, YOU CAN EAT METABOLICALLY HEALTHY ON THESE DIETS

Every one of these diets can offer you significant improvements to your metabolic health. That's because all of these eating plans are better than the SAD. That's not saying much, because the bar is incredibly low. Still, if you're on the SAD like most people, any change is a good change.

The biggest switch is eating whole food. And if you've got easy recipes at hand, you're far more likely to stick to your diet. With that in mind, I've included a few recipes for each eating plan below to help you get started. Just grab the ingredients, throw them in a pan, and you're eating five minutes later.

At the beginning of this chapter, I promised sample meals for each popular diet. Now that you know the good, the bad, and the tasty about each diet, we're ready for those snack and meal ideas. We'll start with carnivore.

A DAY IN THE LIFE OF A METABOLICALLY HEALTHY CARNIVORE

Carnivore meals are a lot simpler and less frequent than you might expect. Most carnivores aren't that hungry because the food is so nutritionally dense and filling. One or two meals a day may be enough to keep you fully satisfied. But the food industry hammers into us the importance of "variety" and "not being bored of the same food" from early childhood. So if you're looking for a little variety in your diet, I'll share a few options for each meal.

Little surprise, the bulk of this diet is meat. Most carnivores eat one to two pounds of meat per day. Because of that, it's hard to overeat, because the protein is so filling. This is the one and only diet on which I can tell you to eat whatever you want within the carnivore diet and just stop eating when you're full. The health and fitness coach P. D. Mangan once wrote, "Nobody binge eats steak." How true that is. Meat has a natural stopping point where you just can't eat any more.

What you do need to watch out for is processed foods. For all of these options, watch the ingredients labels. Many packaged processed meats like bacon have preservatives and chemicals that will hurt your body. That doesn't mean you should just eat raw meat for every meal (please don't try this, no matter what social media carnivores might tell you), but be careful what you're consuming. On the same note, a little salt (electrolytes) is important for all of these foods. Not processed table salt but sea salt or Himalayan salt that retains a wider variety of minerals.

SAMPLE CARNIVORE BREAKFASTS

- Steak and eggs and cheese — For most people, this will be a 6–8 oz. steak and two to three eggs. Pick a healthy cheese that isn't heavily processed and loaded with chemicals.
- Bacon and eggs and cheese — 6–8 oz. of bacon, which is four to six slices, and two to three eggs. Again, pick a smart cheese option.
- A glass of whole milk (optional) or whole milk/heavy cream in your coffee or tea — You may not actually need this because you'll be so full. You may end up drinking a lot of water on this diet because your body just doesn't want the extra calories and fat since it's already so satisfied.

SAMPLE CARNIVORE LUNCHES

- Two hamburger patties with a piece of cheese
- Another 6–8 oz. steak

Need something easy and transportable to take to work? Try fresh sliced chicken or turkey meat and cheese rollups or hard-boiled eggs. Just watch the sliced meat for chemicals and preservatives.

SAMPLE CARNIVORE DINNERS

You might ask, "Carnivores really eat three steaks a day?" Not typically. Then again, some do, depending on their activity level. You may not even want a third meal because you're still so stuffed from all the protein at breakfast and lunch. This makes carnivore easy to pair with intermittent fasting.

If you are going to eat dinner, here are some options:

- 6–8 oz. steak
- Seafood
- 8 oz. of fish with butter

▦ SAMPLE CARNIVORE SNACKS AND DRINKS

Carnivores tend not to snack because they're so loaded down with protein at each meal. That said, some choose not to bulk up on two or three huge meals but might have one big meal and one snack.

The most important consideration isn't how often you eat but making sure you're getting real whole food. Snacks tend to be where most people intake their worst preservatives and chemicals. Be on the lookout for added ingredients like sugar or vegetable and seed oils. If you're going to snack, then snack smart.

- Beef jerky, venison jerky
- Pork rinds
- Cheese
- Fresh sliced chicken or turkey with cheese
- Cream cheese, cottage cheese, yogurt
- Water, coffee, club soda, whole milk

▦ SAMPLE CARNIVORE DESSERTS

- Carnivore cheesecake
- Carnivore pudding — This, like most carnivore desserts, is going to be cream based.

A DAY IN THE LIFE OF A METABOLICALLY HEALTHY GLUTEN-FREE LOW-CARBER

There's a lot more flexibility in this eating plan because the goal is really just to reduce carbs and eliminate gluten. You're not restricted to one type of food. The biggest challenge is avoiding all those replacement options packed with harmful chemicals that will make your body even more sick than it might already be. The good news is that all carnivore options work for this meal plan as well, so you can refer to both meal plan lists.

SAMPLE GLUTEN-FREE, LOW-CARB BREAKFASTS

- Salmon (or bacon) and eggs with a handful of blueberries in plain Greek yogurt and coffee with heavy cream
- Bacon (or salmon) and eggs with a bowl of high-fiber steel-cut oats — The oats give you 23 gm. of carbs. That's about half of the 50 gm. of carbs you can have in a day, so minimize carbs the rest of the day.
- Almond flour pancakes with blueberries or 100 percent dark chocolate chips, topped with butter instead of syrup, and a side of sausage or bacon

SAMPLE GLUTEN-FREE, LOW-CARB LUNCHES

- Turkey and cheese in a lettuce wrap with mayo — Check for non-seed-oil-based mayo, use avocado oil, or make your own from bacon fat.
- Zucchini boat (hollowed out) stuffed with ground sausage and cheese
- Chicken and broccoli stir fry — Make sure to use coconut oil or real olive oil.

A lot of people on this diet prefer a deluxe salad for lunch. This is a great way to get your full nutrition. You can include spinach, cucumbers, tomatoes, avocado, protein (bacon, grilled chicken, or grilled salmon) with a homemade blue cheese dressing. But watch out for preservatives in bottled dressing. Your best bet is to make your own by combining real blue cheese, mayo, sour cream, and whipping cream.

SAMPLE GLUTEN-FREE, LOW-CARB DINNERS

- Spaghetti squash with meatballs and low-sugar tomato sauce — Tomato sauce can come loaded with problems. Make sure you select one with no added sugar and no seed oils or vegetable oils. Eat Happy brand or Rao brand tomato / marinara sauce are good choices. This is not hard to make on your own if you want to be sure.

- Soup — You have a huge range of options here depending on what nutrients you need each day. An easy soup recipe is bone broth, shrimp, chicken, cabbage or spinach, and okra.
- Pho, a Vietnamese dish similar to ramen — Meat (chicken, beef, or pork), bean sprouts, cilantro, mint, mushrooms, bone broth, shirataki noodles (a low-carb noodle substitute)
- Flank steak marinated in lime with guacamole and a side of grilled vegetables — This is a Mexican-style dinner for when you want something different.

SAMPLE GLUTEN-FREE, LOW-CARB SNACKS AND DRINKS

- Low-carb keto substitutes are available for many food options — Look at the ingredients label to confirm they are clean. Beware seed oils, fake sugar substitutes, and sugar alcohols.
- Nuts — Walnuts, pecans, almonds, macadamia nuts. Buy all raw or dry-roasted. Just "roasted" means roasted in seed or vegetable oil.
- Water, coffee, club soda, whole milk — Coffee with heavy cream or coffee with coconut oil (MCT oil). Beware diet soda! It's OK in limited quantities as you're weaning off soda, but evidence shows that sugar substitutes are not great for health long term.
- Organic green tea — There's a big difference between Lipton and loose-leaf teas, not only for health but for flavor. Experiment with better quality and see the difference for yourself.
- Kombucha (a fermented beverage with positive microbiome influence)

▨ SAMPLE GLUTEN-FREE, LOW-CARB DESSERTS

- Low-carb keto substitutes available — Look at the ingredients label to confirm they are clean. Beware seed oils, fake sugar substitutes, and sugar alcohols. Rosette's brand is safe.
- Fat bombs — Combine coconut oil, peanut butter (no sugar added), and cocoa powder (100 percent), then put them on a sheet of wax paper and freeze them. They're great during a hot day.
- Homemade ice cream — This may sound intimidating, but it's easy to make and fun for the whole family. It's just whole milk, heavy cream, ice, vanilla, and stevia. You can top it with a whole mint leaf for aesthetics and flavor. Look up a recipe online and enjoy the experience.

A DAY IN THE LIFE OF A METABOLICALLY HEALTHY MEDITERRANEAN DIETER

In some ways, the Mediterranean diet is the easiest to follow. It's not as concerned with carb counting as it is with living a generally more wholesome lifestyle. You're supposed to walk, spend more time with the people you love, and eat smaller portions of leaner foods. As such, many of these meal options can be made in larger portions to be shared at a table with family and friends.

The biggest difference between Mediterranean and low-carb is more beans, potatoes, whole grain bread, whole grain pastas, and way more seafood and fish. This diet is easier if you live somewhere with access to cheap and fresh fish so you're not paying a fortune for frozen ingredients that might not taste as good.

Notice how often olive oil is used. Make sure you're buying clean and pure olive oil from a source you trust. If you use inferior olive oil every time with seed oils mixed in, you're going to be damaging your body even as you think you're getting healthy. Don't shy away from paying a little extra to make sure your olive oil is fostering the metabolic health you need for a long life.

SAMPLE MEDITERRANEAN BREAKFASTS

- Low-sugar Greek yogurt with berries and nuts mixed in, plus an omelet with vegetables (onions, mushrooms, spinach)
- Low-carb gluten-free oatmeal with raisins
- Gluten-free lavash (no seed or vegetable oils added) with cream cheese, tomato, fresh sliced chicken or turkey, and real olive oil

SAMPLE MEDITERRANEAN LUNCHES

- Gluten-free lavash (no seed or vegetable oils added) with hummus (no seed or vegetable oils added) and olive oil
- Salad with goat cheese, shrimp, lettuce, garbanzo beans, olive oil, and a little vinaigrette

SAMPLE MEDITERRANEAN DINNERS

- Salmon with olive oil and eggplant fries (air fried with olive oil)
- Chicken and vegetable stir fry in olive oil
- Grilled shrimp with sautéed kale in olive oil

SAMPLE MEDITERRANEAN SNACKS AND DRINKS

- Sliced veggies with hummus
- Olives and cheese (mixed together like a salad-like dish)
- Red wine (dryer red wine like merlot or cabernet)

SAMPLE MEDITERRANEAN DESSERTS

- Plain Greek yogurt with tablespoon of honey
- Baklava (once or twice a year for me)
- Turkish delight (once or twice a year for me)

A DAY IN THE LIFE OF A METABOLICALLY HEALTHY VEGAN

The major challenge with plant-based diets is getting enough nutrition from a variety of plant sources and supplements. In particular, protein can be a major challenge to those who don't prepare in advance. Beans and peas are how most vegans get the bulk of their protein.

There are a lot of products advertised to the vegan community. Most of these are packed with seed and vegetable oils. Beware chemical slop with a "vegan" or "plant-based" label. For example, cancer-causing glyphosate is technically "vegan" but appears in some brands of advertised nondairy milk. Another example, "JUST Egg," has corn starch, canola oil, and twelve chemicals in the ingredients. Avoid this product like the plague—the perfect metaphor for the immunity-weakening effect of its ultraprocessed ingredients. At least highly publicized meat substitute brand Impossible is accurately named. It's impossible for this food product to support your metabolic health.

If you're going to stick to the vegan diet, be smart and educate yourself about your body's needs, the foods you're eating, and what nutrition you'll need long term. Dr. Casey Means offered the sample meal suggestions you're about to read. In addition to real, whole, plant-based food, Dr. Means supplements her diet with 3,000mg EPA/DHA, B12, and a daily multivitamin.

▦ SAMPLE VEGAN BREAKFASTS

Many vegans enjoy a green smoothie for breakfast. You can enjoy it on the go, and it won't leave you feeling bloated or weighed down through the rest of your morning. A green smoothie usually includes:

- Low-carb, no-added-sugar, high-protein powder / shake (2 carbs per serving) — You can find these at Whole Foods and other health-food stores as well as online.
- 3 cups of greens (spinach, kale, or mix)
- 2 tbsp. of chia seeds or flaxseeds (organic)

- Half a cup of walnuts
- 1 tbsp. organic prebiotic fiber
- 1 scoop of greens powder (wheatgrass, etc.)
- Half-handful of frozen mixed berries
- Water

Metabolically healthy breakfasts Dr. Means enjoys include:

- Chia pudding with coconut milk, almond butter, lime juice, walnuts, and a few berries
- Tofu scramble (tofu, nutritional yeast, black salt) with a ton of veggies
- Almond flour pancakes with a few berries.
- Tofu quiche with crust made from almond flour or grain-free cauliflower pizza crusts (no seed oils)

▨ SAMPLE VEGAN LUNCHES

- Can of organic beans (40g protein) on a big salad with bell peppers, tomatoes, onions, kale, arugula, capers, sauerkraut, walnuts, pumpkin seeds, chia seeds, and dressing of tahini and liquid aminos and apple cider vinegar
- Collard green wrap filled with hummus, avocado, tofu, veggies
- Veggie stir fry with beans or tofu over cauliflower rice
- Many different soups (lentil soup, etc)
- Tacos made with mushroom and walnut or cauliflower and walnut baked "taco meat" filled with veggies, cashew crema, in a butter lettuce "taco shell," flax tortilla, or jicama tortilla

▨ SAMPLE VEGAN DINNERS

- Bag of frozen organic cauliflower rice with tofu, a bunch of veggies, tamari, almond butter, etc, for a sort of asian/pad thai-esq stir fry

- Zucchini noodles with pesto made from arugula, walnuts, salt, nutritional yeast.
- Cauliflower pizza crust with veggies and homemade tomato sauce and almond parmesan (almonds, salt, nutritional yeast in the food processor) or other nut-based sauce (blended) with nuts, water, olive oil, spices, tamari
- Lentil curry over cauliflower rice
- Cauliflower rice sushi filled with avocado and veggies (takes ten minutes to make)
- Homemade black bean and flax burger in a lettuce wrap with Primal Kitchen's sugar-free ketchup

SAMPLE VEGAN SNACKS AND DRINKS

- Avocado
- Olives
- Nuts and seeds
- Apples or pears (both don't spike many people's glucose) with almond butter and chia seeds
- Romaine hearts or flax seed crackers dipped in hummus or olive tapenade.
- Mushroom jerky (no sugar added, low seed and vegetable oils)
- Dairy milk alternative beverages — Watch out for seed and vegetable oils!
- Homemade nut-based cheeses and milk alternatives

SAMPLE VEGAN DESSERTS

As with other dietary plans, homemade always beats store bought. This is especially true with the vegan diet because making it yourself prevents any animal products from accidentally making their way into your food without your knowledge. You never have to wonder when you've added each ingredient yourself.

- Black bean brownies with allulose or dates
- Chickpea cookie dough sweetened with a couple dates and chopped 88 percent chocolate
- Chocolate and avocado pudding
- Almond flour cake with coconut oil and cocoa icing
- Chocolate chia pudding
- Strawberries dipped in melted 90 percent dark chocolate
- Fat bombs — Coconut oil, peanut butter (no sugar added), and cocoa powder (100 percent). Place these on wax paper and freeze them for a great summer treat.

WHERE TO NEXT?

If you're like me when I read, you've been taking notes and snapping pictures of the meal and snack lists that most align with your preferences. Your next grocery order will be one to remember.

As you buy and prepare new and likely familiar foods, keep the first metabolic health principle in mind: **a system, not a goal**. I recommend eating the suggested meals based on your preferred diet. That doesn't mean never try anything new. I could eat steak and eggs for breakfast every morning for the rest of my life because I like the high-protein routine. Some people need variety. And that's OK.

Treat these sample meals as training. You're learning what serves your body's needs and what doesn't. Whether you're gluten-free or vegan (or both), you'll be able to assemble metabolically healthy ingredients that make a tasty, nutritious meal.

While you're enjoying your next metabolically healthy meal, let's give you some further reading. The one topic we haven't yet covered in this book is simply called "miscellaneous." Over the years as a cardiac surgeon and now as a private practice metabolic health specialist, I've heard every question and concern about heart health, dietary choices, and everything else that affects both. So before we close out this book, I'm going to share with you my answers to the most frequently asked (and also rarely answered) questions pertaining to your metabolic health. Let's go.

FREQUENTLY ASKED, RARELY ANSWERED QUESTIONS ABOUT METABOLIC HEALTH

Now that you've read most of this book, I expect you have a lot of questions. You just learned that you've been fed a steady diet of half-truths and outright lies all your life. You need answers, and you need them now.

I sympathize with your urgency. I felt the same when I learned the truth about metabolic health. No one wants to be left in the dark when it comes to how to avoid a painful and early death. And I'm glad you're hungry for answers. That means you're taking your health seriously, you're not content to leave it in the hands of uneducated doctors, and you're going to push through the food industry's lies until you find the truth.

Most clients I counsel come back to our second session with a dozen burning questions. And even more people write to me on social media and private forums looking for answers. The frequent recurrence of many of those questions indicates a need for definitive answers that align with the seven metabolic health principles.

I've compiled a list of those answers in this chapter. The topics discussed herein will help guide the further research you'll want to do after finishing this book. Some questions and my answers will repeat or at least rhyme with material you've read so far. I'm all right with that because at least a few readers will skip all previous seven chapters and come straight here. I don't want you to miss anything important.

One more quick note before you begin the FAQs. I've left references to me, Dr. Philip Ovadia, in several questions where my views were directly asked for. Since you've read this far in your book, I take it that you, too, are curious about my thoughts on these topics.

GENERAL METABOLIC HEALTH FAQ

WHAT IS METABOLIC HEALTH?

You'll want to explain what you've learned in this book to family, friends, and coworkers. A concise definition of metabolic health will help you teach others, so I'll sum it up in three sentences.

Metabolic health refers to the body's ability to properly use food for fuel, growth, and repair, and to store energy for periods of lower food availability. Loss of metabolic health leads to many chronic diseases such as type 2 diabetes, high blood pressure, obesity, heart disease, fatty liver disease, gallstones, polycystic ovarian syndrome (PCOS), obstructive sleep apnea, gout, and more.[45] Markers of metabolic health include waist circumference, blood pressure, HDL cholesterol, triglycerides, and fasting glucose.

SHOULDN'T I JUST EXERCISE MORE?

Yes, you should exercise. But you can't out-exercise a bad diet.

The primary goal of exercise should be to build and maintain muscle. Because muscle is more metabolically active, more muscle keeps you healthier. To that end, being more active throughout the day is more effective than isolated bursts of exercise amid long periods of inactivity.

---

45 Katie McCallum, "What Is Metabolic Syndrome & Can It Be Reversed?" On Health, Houston Methodist, last updated April 5, 2021, https://www.houstonmethodist.org/blog/articles/2021/apr/what-is-metabolic-syndrome-and-can-it-be-reversed/.

Translation: Instead of hitting the gym three times a week, find ways to build more activity into your daily life. You'll feel better in the short term as your body bulks up, and your long-term health will be stronger because you've improved your metabolic processing.

WHAT ARE THE SIMPLEST CHANGES THAT HAVE THE BIGGEST METABOLIC HEALTH IMPACT?

I'll give you five changes you can start right now that will get you rolling with the biggest payoff:

- Eat real whole food
- Eliminate processed fats (vegetable/seed oils)
- Minimize added sugars and processed carbs
- Get adequate amounts of quality sleep
- Move more

If you start doing those five things right now and stay consistent for six months, you'll see unbelievable results. All the other changes in this book can layer on top of these initial changes to create even greater impact.

HOW SHOULD I TRACK METABOLIC HEALTH?

I encourage my clients to use four specific tracking methods.

The first two metrics are waist circumference and body fat percentage. These are great external markers you can measure. Most people can rely on these metrics to start with, but they're not perfect. As we've discussed, some people can look healthy on the outside but have metabolic problems on the inside.

Third, to dive deeper into real metabolic health, get some blood work done. Specifically your insulin level, fasting glucose level, and a cholesterol panel (checking your low-triglyceride, high-HDL ratio). Finally, monitor your blood pressure, since that's a great marker for how your heart is doing. Also, if you can locate one, a continuous glucose monitor will help you figure out which carbs are better or worse for your body to consume.

WHAT ARE HIDDEN RISKS THAT "HEALTHY" BUT INACTIVE PEOPLE FACE?

What is your definition of "healthy?" If you just mean "not obese," that's not metabolic health. A person can be skinny on the outside and still have overweight symptoms on the inside. It's called "skinny fat." I've operated on plenty of those people.

And "healthy" food isn't actually healthy. Vegetable oils are clearly not healthy. The salad dressings most "healthy people" eat are loaded with high-fructose corn syrup. And low-fat "diet" snacks are high-carb processed crap.

So let's set aside the *appearance* of health. If you're looking for real health, it's going to require activity. It's hard for inactive people to be healthy because they don't have as much muscle and don't burn as much energy. It's more likely the food they eat will end up in fat storage as opposed to energy or muscle.

If you want real health instead of just the appearance of health, you're going to need to include some physical activity in your daily life.

IS HAVING GAS A SIGN OF POOR METABOLIC HEALTH?

Some gas is normal. Significant gas issues could indicate inflammation in the GI tract, leading to bloating. If you're frequently bloated or passing gas, you could have a dietary issue.

WHAT EFFECT DOES METABOLIC HEALTH HAVE ON DEGENERATIVE DISEASE?

Degenerative diseases are metabolic diseases. Fix your metabolic health, and your risk for these issues drop to nearly zero, barring extremely rare conditions. And even in those rare circumstances, better metabolic health will help improve your quality of life.

WHAT'S THE EFFECT OF SAUNA ON METABOLIC HEALTH?

Sauna is said to be beneficial to metabolic health, which may have to do with the direct physiological effects along with mental health and stress relief habits.[46] It's worth doing some research if you're interested in this topic.

HOW DO YOU WAKE YOUR METABOLISM UP SAFELY AFTER BEING SEDENTARY AND OUT OF SHAPE FOR A LONG TIME?

First, improve your diet from a metabolic standpoint. That will take some weight off and give you more energy. Then increase your physical activities, which doesn't mean going to the gym. It means taking the stairs, getting a standing desk, and other small daily changes that add a little more effort and a little more muscle growth.

These are easy changes anyone can make even under extreme metabolic sickness.

ADVICE FOR PEOPLE WITH A SLOW METABOLISM?

Read this book. Then read it again. ☺

On a serious note now, muscle is the most metabolically active tissue.[47] The more you build, the more you can increase your metabolism. A slow metabolism could be a sign of insufficient muscle density to warrant a high level of energy burn, so your body doesn't bother stoking the furnace any hotter than it has to. Why work harder than necessary, right?

In that case, it's less that you have a slow or poor metabolism and more a matter of, "Stop damaging your metabolism." Your natural metabolism will return once you build muscle and clean the toxins out of your diet.

---

46 Kimberly Truong, "The Infrared Sauna Is Not a Weight Loss Tool," Vice, last updated January 10, 2019, https://www.vice.com/en/article/bje9gv/the-infrared-sauna-is-not-a-weight-loss-tool

47 "MUSCLE BOUND: Muscle is metabolically active, fat-burning . . ." Chicago Tribune, last updated April 12, 1995, https://www.chicagotribune.com/news/ct-xpm-1995-04-12-9504130151-story.html#:~:text=MUSCLE%20BOUND%3A%20Muscle%20is%20metabolically%20active%2C%20fat%2Dburning%20tissue,need%20more%20calories%20for%20support.

ON AVERAGE I SLEEP ABOUT FIVE HOURS A NIGHT, AND I KNOW I SHOULD BE SLEEPING MORE. WHAT IMPACT DOES LACK OF SLEEP HAVE ON METABOLIC HEALTH?

Lack of sleep stresses the body. Stress has a major impact on your metabolic health. And it's not just the amount of sleep, it's the quality.

Improving your sleep quality is a virtuous cycle. Sleeping better will improve your metabolic health. Improving your metabolic health means your sleep quality improves further, and you may not need as much sleep to function optimally.

Get more sleep, and get better sleep. This is foundational to good health.

WHAT ARE SOME SIGNS OF SUCCESS WHEN DEVELOPING HEALTHIER DIETARY HABITS?

Track your metabolic health improvement according to the measurements I included above and in the chapter on tracking metabolic health. That includes external signs like waist circumference and body fat percentage but also internal measurements like blood sugar and blood pressure.

On a day-to-day basis you can also focus on your energy levels. Better metabolic health will give you a lot more good days than bad days.

WHAT ARE SOME SUGGESTIONS ON MAINTAINING CONSTANT ENERGY THROUGHOUT THE DAY INSTEAD OF COMING UP HARD AND DOWN HARD?

The energy yo-yo is the result of too much sugar. Our bodies aren't meant for the levels of sugar we take in, and they crash when that huge influx of chemicals runs out. It's not natural.

As your metabolism improves, your body will use fat as fuel instead of sugar. And your body will process sugar differently than it does now. You won't crave it as much, and you won't be constantly riding the sugar roller-coaster.

HOW MUCH OF SOMEONE'S METABOLIC HEALTH IS GENETIC VERSUS HABIT AND LIFESTYLE?

When we look at family heart disease, obesity and poor metabolic health tend to run in those same families. That's interpreted as genetic. In reality, it's environmental. My parents were obese, and so was I. I believed it was genetic until I realized we were eating the same wrong foods.

In my experience, only about 5 percent of metabolic syndrome cases are genetic. That means 95 percent are environmental, i.e., your diet and fitness choices. Before you decide genetics are your issue and there's no point in trying to get better, adjust your food and exercise.

WHAT IS THE NUMBER ONE STEP A YOUNG, HEALTHY PERSON SHOULD TAKE TO ENSURE GREAT METABOLIC HEALTH?

Eat real whole food. This is always the first answer.

A close second is to think long term about your health and food habits. Better to develop these early and make them "normal" for you rather than fall off and have to completely change later in adulthood like I did.

WHAT IS THE BEST WAY TO IMPROVE METABOLIC HEALTH ON A BUDGET?

Stick to real whole food. You'll be less hungry, eat less overall, and waste much less food. For example, with my carnivore diet, I waste nothing, not even fat from the meat because I can use it in cooking. Meat doesn't spoil quickly. Shopping for carnivores is easier and cheaper than for people eating the Standard American Diet.

Cheap ground beef is still way better quality food than anything out of a box. Organ meats are also inexpensive because they are low demand. Look at the nutritional impact of beef liver. It's one of the most cost-effective foods you can eat. So are eggs.

After the second COVID-19 relief payment in the US, I tweeted: "For about $600 you can eat two pounds of ground beef and a few eggs a day for the next ninety days. Pair it with some body weight resistance training (free). By Tax Day you will improve your metabolic health, have a lower chance of getting ill from viruses, and feel much better overall."

Cheap processed foods cost us more because we need more to feel satiated. But you can eat extremely well on a limited budget.

▦ HOW DOES METABOLIC HEALTH INTERSECT WITH FATTY LIVER?

In my experience, the primary cause of liver disease I observe is no longer alcohol; it's fatty liver. That's a diet-related condition. Therefore, your metabolic health directly correlates to the most common liver disease. Cleaning up your metabolic health can heal your liver.

FOOD AND DIET FAQ

▦ WHERE DO I BUY REAL WHOLE FOOD?

Shop local. This goes for carnivores, vegans, and everyone in between. Talk to the farmers in your area; gardeners and ranchers, too. You'd be shocked how many of them offer direct sales of products at much cheaper prices than you'd pay at the grocery store. The trade-off is that you might need to buy in larger quantities to make it worth their while. They typically don't want to sell you just enough for a meal or two. That might mean you buy half a cow, get it processed, and put it in your freezer.

For carnivores, go to **meatrx.com** to look up local ranchers. Omnivores and our vegetarian friends should try **eatlocal.com**. You likely have a lot more local options than you realize. For those living in cities, a local provider might be just a thirty-minute drive away. These are great alternatives.

Remember that it's better to build up your community than invest in Big Agriculture. That ensures you get fresh ingredients you can trust, and your food hasn't been processed in huge factories and loaded with chemicals.

If all else fails, you can still find real whole food in most grocery stores. That just requires you to buy basics like meat and vegetables and do the cooking yourself. However, most supermarket food isn't as nutrient dense as the products you'd get from a local supplier. Whenever possible, stick with the locals.

▧ DOES EATING CARNIVORE DAMAGE MY HEALTH IN THE LONG RUN?

Any way of eating can be damaging if too much processed food is incorporated. For carnivores, this would include things like lunch meats and hot dogs. That's the sort of diet most people imagine when they think of carnivores.

But if you're eating a proper carnivore diet that gives you the full nutritional balance a human body requires, there is absolutely zero evidence of long-term harm. Historical and modern populations throughout the world, like the Inuit tribes, have lived on carnivore diets.

And a mostly carnivore diet was good enough for the human race during our extensive evolution. We didn't have agriculture until about ten thousand years ago, and we only invented grocery stores relatively recently. A carnivore diet was good enough for our ancestors.

▧ IF I AM GOING TO EAT CARBS, WHICH ONES ARE PREFERABLE?

The less processed, the better. Avoid processed foods like snack chips. You can eat a baked potato, raw honey, or steel-cut oats instead.

▧ HOW CLOSELY DO I NEED TO MONITOR MY CALORIC INTAKE, ASSUMING I'M EATING FEWER THAN 50 GRAMS OF CARBS A DAY?

It's hard to determine how many calories you are eating and burning each day. What you eat affects how much you burn, as well. It's enough to make your head spin, and learning to count calories can present a high mental barrier to people trying to become healthy.

In general, I do not tell people to focus on calories. I tell them to eat high-quality foods until they are full and to eat only when they are hungry. Yes, you will need fewer calories in than out to lose weight, but focusing on how many calories is the wrong approach. Tracking the type of food you eat is a better approach, together with eating only when hungry and stopping when full. That way your body gets what it needs without going to excess, and you can be sure you're getting clean fuel instead of polluted toxins.

HOW DO I INCREASE PROTEIN INTAKE WITHOUT INCREASING CALORIES?

Most protein we eat goes to building and rebuilding tissue, particularly muscles. Protein overconsumption studies show that if you eat excessive protein without excess carb intake, you will not get fat. In fact, some nutrition experts say that protein should not really count as calories. I'm talking specifically about real whole-food protein.

You can't really eat excessive amounts of unprocessed proteins, particularly animal proteins. It's just about impossible to eat 5,000 calories' worth of steak. Most people will hit a wall and not be able to eat another bite.

Finally, a high-protein diet will replace most other sources of calories. More meat means less room for potato chips and cookies. That's a huge benefit if temptation is an issue early in your metabolic health journey.

WHAT IS DR. OVADIA'S OPINION ON INTERMITTENT FASTING?

IF is a great tool for improving metabolic health.

The damage bad food does to our metabolic health depends on (1) what we eat and (2) how often we eat. We eat so much more often than our ancestors or even grandparents did. We must allow our bodies to be in recovery mode after eating. After a meal, especially a high-carb meal, it takes about four to six hours for our insulin levels to return to base levels. Most people eat three meals and three snacks a day, so most people's insulin levels never come down, so they are constantly elevated—and driving toward insulin resistance. A simple daily sixteen-hour fast allows your body to rest. Even if you are on a high-carb diet, this improves your metabolic health.

The only downside of this high-carb diet is the body's reliance on glucose as a fuel source. As soon as your sugar levels drop, your body sends hunger signals, so it becomes harder to fast. This can change as you adopt a better diet, but there's an adjustment period. I tell people changing from high-carb to low-carb diets to not worry about fasting for two to three weeks. Once they get fat adapted and into ketosis, they naturally start fasting because they're hungry less often.

As for me, I don't force myself to fast. I let it occur naturally. Because when I eat right, I'm less hungry less often. Eating enough protein and fat to stay satiated means I'm not hungry all the time. So I fast intermittently without thinking about it.

WHAT IS PHILIP'S TAKE ON DAIRY FOR THOSE WHO HAVE NO ISSUE WITH IT? IS DAIRY AS BAD AS GLUTEN? DOES SOMEONE WHO STOPS EATING MILK AND YOGURT BUT CONSUMES OTHER DAIRY PRODUCTS FARE BETTER?

I have no issues with dairy because it's a real whole food. It's fat, protein, and a host of nutrients. And it kept our ancestors alive when other food was scarce.

That said, I believe dairy should be consumed as close to its real form as possible. That means no skim milk or added sugar and carbs. Eat real cheese, not cheese-like processed products like single American slices from the grocery. That's basically plastic flavored like cheese, and it's not good for you.

Dairy has been improperly implicated as bad for our health. It's high in fat, and fat was the scapegoat the food industry needed to take pressure off sugar. For a while, eggs were also supposedly killing us. Now it's meat. None of these are as addictive as sugar, which means the food industry would rather you skip them and go for the moneymaking products they can produce for cheap. Their profits go up. If that kills you in the process, they can always find more consumers.

Remember this simple maxim: **If your ancestors ate it, it's probably good for you. If scientists invented it in the twentieth century or later, it's probably poison.**

■ IS EXCESSIVE PROTEIN BAD FOR YOUR KIDNEYS?

Someone once asked me a way more detailed version of this question: "How accurate are creatinine levels for determining estimated glomerular filtration rate (eGFR) in a fit and muscular man?" They boil down to about the same thing, so I can answer both by answering the complicated version.

The higher your creatinine level, and the lower your eGFR, the worse your kidney function is. However, if you are eating a lot of protein, you may have higher creatinine, which does not correlate with kidney issues on its own. You also need to monitor that eGFR level or check a cystatin C level, which operates independently from consuming protein.

This is another case of assuming something is bad because of correlation, like blaming cholesterol for heart attacks when it's really the damage caused by blood sugar that creates the cholesterol problem. In actuality, there is adequate research to suggest that a high protein intake improves kidney function.

■ WHAT FOODS INCREASE YOUR METABOLISM?

Flip that around. There are clearly foods that *damage* your metabolism. Don't eat those, and your metabolism will increase to its natural level. As for naturally increasing your metabolism, focus on building muscle. That improves your metabolism. Combine these two processes to boost your metabolism. That's the best method according to all the research.

■ WHAT ALTERNATIVES TO CARBOHYDRATE ENERGY DRINKS CAN LONG-DISTANCE RUNNERS USE?

When you're on a high-carb diet, your body fuels itself with carbs, especially sugar. Once you're in ketosis, you become fat adapted, meaning you've trained your body to use fat as energy. Your body can use its own fat, which is great for slimming down. Or you can eat fat. Or drink it.

A product called UltraFat works great for runners. It fuels your body with fat instead of carbs, so you don't get the blood sugar rise and crash. Plus, your workout will be less prone to cause food binges later because you aren't burning off temporary fuel; you're harnessing more natural energy. You can find UltraFat in stores or online, including on Amazon.

IS IT NECESSARY TO RAISE CHILDREN ON A LOW-CARB DIET, OR DO THEY NEED MORE CARBS FOR PROPER GROWTH?

Children do not need carbs to grow. Because children are actively growing, they have a greater carb threshold. That means they can safely eat more carbs, but they needn't necessarily do so.

Instead of restricting their diets, focus on teaching them the most important habits: eating real whole food and avoiding processed carbs and seed/vegetable oils. Get them used to eating good food and avoiding poison. They'll see the difference in high school when they're fitter and happier than their metabolically unhealthy peers.

SUPPLEMENTS FAQ

ARE SUPPLEMENTS THE ONLY WAY TO MAINTAIN METABOLIC HEALTH?

No. If you're eating right, you likely won't need supplements at all, unless there's something wrong with your food or your body. We discussed the soil issue earlier, but other specific concerns might exist.

Our ancestors didn't evolve using supplements. We don't need them, either. Don't just mindlessly take supplements. Only take them if you have measurable deficiencies after eating real whole food or if your body isn't processing the nutrients for some reason.

WHAT ARE THE BEST SUPPLEMENTS TO REDUCE BLOOD PRESSURE?

The best way to have normal blood pressure is good metabolic health with a good diet. You should not need supplements. High blood pressure is usually the earliest warning sign of poor metabolic health. Rarely is high BP caused by anything else.

Treating high BP is like silencing a warning signal. Physicians and the systems treat high BP as a normal thing that happens as you age, when it is not. It's a loud alarm that something is wrong in your body and you need to address it before it kills you. If you have high BP, you need to investigate and correct it.

SHOULD I TAKE A MAGNESIUM SUPPLEMENT?

Our food supply is generally magnesium deficient. That's bad news because magnesium is important for a range of crucial biological processes in our bodies. It's key for all of our organ functions up to and including bone growth. Magnesium deficiency can contribute to heart problems, as well as sleep, energy, and other health issues.

We're supposed to get magnesium from our diets, especially from leafy green vegetables (or from the meat of animals that eat leafy green vegetables). But poor soil quality lowers magnesium across the entire food chain. A well-rounded whole-food diet maximizes your chances of not being magnesium deficient, but soil issues may still cause deficiency.

If you're deficient, magnesium supplements can be useful, but be aware of possible side effects. Magnesium sulfate and citrate are used as bowel-cleansing agents. In high doses, they cause unpleasant side effects. Magnesium glycinate is the best tolerated in your body, or you can use full-spectrum magnesium. I don't personally endorse one form over another. It's all about how much you can take without loose bowel movements.

If you're going to take magnesium supplements, and research does indicate they can be helpful, experiment until you find one that gives you the benefits without the digestive drawbacks.

WHAT IS DR. OVADIA'S OPINION ON PREWORKOUT SUPPLEMENTS LIKE ARGININE, CARNITINE, AND CITRULLINE?

In general, I prefer people to get all the nutrients they need from their diet as opposed to supplements. Eating a healthy diet, which means mostly protein and fat, largely makes supplementation unnecessary. Avoid paying a bunch of money for supplements you don't need and won't benefit from.

MEDICATIONS FAQ

I'M ON THREE BLOOD PRESSURE MEDICATIONS AND HAVE A FAMILY HISTORY OF STROKE. I'VE STOPPED TAKING STATINS. IS THAT OK? SHOULD I RESUME THE MEDICATION?

This book is not medical advice. That includes my answer to this question. I am not here to tell people not to take their medication or to get on new medication. Those choices need to be made personally between you and a competent, educated doctor who understands your specific medical health.

That said, consider the real causes of high blood pressure, stroke, and heart disease. They are all symptoms of metabolic health issues! Often, I have found that when people get their metabolic health in proper shape, they no longer need medication. Real whole food reverses the diseases their medications were prescribed to treat. But many choose to continue to use their medication as they work toward health just to prevent any complications from symptoms.

The bottom line about medications is that you need to be working with a knowledgeable physician who understands metabolic health. Otherwise you may just be treating symptoms and ignoring the real danger. If you cannot find one locally, visit **ovadiahearthealth.com**.

I HAVE FAMILIAL HYPERCHOLESTEROLEMIA (FH). DO I NEED A STATIN?

It's not clear that elevated cholesterol causes heart attacks. It's the blood clotting. That being the case, the presence of FH doesn't change my metabolic health recommendations. Patients with FH may need to be more aggressive with elevated cholesterol levels, and that might include pharmaceutical therapies in addition to improving your metabolic health. That way, you address immediate symptoms while still planning for long-term health.

You need a knowledgeable physician. Most will give you the medication and call it a day. They may even resist some of the nutrition changes you want to make. If you've got FH, it's incredibly important to find a doctor who will work with you on this journey.

WHO CAN BENEFIT FROM STATINS, IF ANYONE?

Statins can benefit people who have already had a heart attack or have stents. It's not necessarily for people trying to prevent the first event, only people at risk for a second event. The best prevention for the first event is to get your metabolic health under control. That's also the best prevention for the second event.

But if your metabolic health is dangerously poor, and if you're at high risk, statins can help control the risks as you get yourself into better shape and out of the danger zone.

HORMONAL HEALTH FAQ

CAN I INCREASE TESTOSTERONE WITHOUT TRT?

Yes, you can increase your testosterone without testosterone replacement therapy (TRT). Testosterone deficiency is usually due to poor metabolic health. We know that men's T levels have decreased over the past fifty years, and that decrease corresponds with a massively increased incidence of poor metabolic health.

On a personal note, when I improved my metabolic health, my T levels went up. Way up.

Low T doesn't automatically require treatment with TRT. You need to find the root cause, which is often metabolic health. Building muscle is one major way to raise your testosterone. A real whole food diet and the exercise program in this book lead to more lean mass and less fat mass. All of these changes could mean massive T gains. I recommend giving them a try before using something as drastic as TRT to address what could be a metabolic issue.

▦ WILL IMPROVING METABOLIC HEALTH IMPROVE MY SEX LIFE?

Most definitely. Metabolic health is hormonal health. This includes T levels for men and estrogen for women. Erectile dysfunction in particular is a symptom of poor metabolic health. And once you've shed the fat, your body will be leaner, look better, and respond faster. Those are all excellent benefits when it comes to sexual satisfaction. In short, eat better, love better.

HOW MUCH DOES METABOLIC HEALTH PLAY INTO MAINTAINING HORMONE BALANCE AS WOMEN AGE? CAN BEING METABOLICALLY HEALTHY FIX HORMONE IMBALANCE DURING PERIMENOPAUSE AND MENOPAUSE?

Research shows positive improvement in all of the above conditions when metabolic health improves. Fixing a bad diet fixes the hormone problems that spring from it.

In a perfect world, metabolic health should come before any other treatment option like hormone replacement. TRT carries many potential long-term side effects that can be avoided by fixing your metabolism instead. If you struggle with hormone issues, and if you're worried about your hormones as you age, your best option is to get metabolically healthy now and see how your body responds when it's doing what nature designed it to do.

HEART ISSUES FAQ

▦ DOESN'T CHOLESTEROL CAUSE HEART DISEASE?

High LDL cholesterol is not the root cause of heart disease. In the setting of poor metabolic health, LDL cholesterol may become oxidized (damaged) and contribute to the process that leads to heart disease. Many people that develop heart disease do not have high LDL cholesterol.

Having high triglycerides and low HDL cholesterol are more powerful risk markers for heart disease than having high LDL cholesterol. Damage to the blood vessels of the heart due to inflammation, smoking, and high blood sugar occurs prior to cholesterol accumulation that causes blockages in the arteries. Then doctors see cholesterol blockages and blame the cholesterol.

In the same way that getting shot leads to blood loss, you could claim that some cholesterol causes heart disease. In this case, the bullet is usually high blood sugar. Cholesterol becomes a problem as a result of that initial stress on your body. Fix your metabolic health, and cholesterol ceases to be a problem.

HOW DO RESTING HEART RATE AND BLOOD PRESSURE RELATE?

Resting heart rate is usually a good measure of overall health. Blood pressure usually is, too. The two are not necessarily related to each other. One is a direct indicator; the other is an indirect indicator. Both can be improved with metabolic health.

HOW CAN SOMEONE SAFELY IMPLEMENT A KETO OR LOW-CARB DIET AFTER A HEART ATTACK?

None of the seven principles of metabolic health change if you've had a heart attack. But seven of the ten top causes of death are poor metabolic health, so getting metabolic health under control is your best bet if you want to prevent another heart attack.

Changing your diet after a heart attack can be scary because you aren't sure how your body is going to react. Many doctors will recommend dropping your fat and salt intake to dangerously low levels. But you don't have to do low-fat keto, because real fat doesn't cause heart attacks.

Remember how we discussed that cholesterol blockages come from damage caused by sugar? It's sugar you need to avoid. Stop the damage, and the cholesterol won't build up anymore. You'll halt your increasing risk of damage and will give your body time to heal. That's one of the best steps you can take if you've already had a heart attack.

WHAT ARE THE DIETARY CONSIDERATIONS FOR THOSE WHO ALREADY HAVE HEART DAMAGE DUE TO CHEMO AND RADIATION THERAPY?

Existing damage from chemo and radiation does not change my general recommendations. This type of damage is all the more reason to address your metabolic health and prevent further damage to your heart.

If you're worried you've diminished your lifespan, get control of your metabolic health and maximize your heart's health.

AS A MAN WHO HAS HAD TWO HEART ATTACKS AND NOW HAS EIGHT STENTS, I WONDER WHAT EVIDENCE SHOWS THAT MY STRICT KETO DIET IS REVERSING MY CORONARY ARTERY DISEASE.

You need to work with a physician who knows about both heart health and metabolic health. Advanced testing and imaging of the heart and the blood vessels will likely be required to determine not only your existing damage but also the reversal your better diet is creating. CAT scans or angiograms might also be necessary.

If you're looking for a physician knowledgeable about heart health and metabolic health, Ovadia Heart Health is ready to help you. And if you want someone local, get in touch with me, and I'll do my best to help you find someone closer to your area.

WHAT ARE DR. OVADIA'S VIEWS ON CORONARY ARTERY CALCIUM SCANS AND REVERSAL OF EXISTING CALCIFICATION ON A KETOGENIC DIET?

I think that coronary artery calcium scoring (CACS), also called a coronary calcium scan, is a highly underutilized tool. I'm a big fan of CACS because it looks at the actual disease in the heart instead of trying to imply risk of disease based on blood markers. I also think the test is underutilized in terms of disease reversal.

The CAC scan looks for calcium in the arteries of the heart and assigns a score based on how much calcium is present. If you score zero, I would say you only have about a 1 percent chance of developing heart disease over the following five to ten years. That's what everyone should hope for.

Scoring more than zero puts you at a certain risk of heart disease, depending on your age. On average, CAC scores in people with heart disease will go up 10 to 20 percent per year, based on my experience. Progressing slower than that puts you into a low-risk category.

Unfortunately, no intervention has currently been shown to reliably reverse calcification. Yes, there have been some reversals, but as of now we don't have a reliable method to replicate it for everyone. I tell my clients that we're not necessarily looking for reversal. We're really just looking to stop progression. Maintaining good metabolic health after halting CAC progression cuts your risk and diminishes the threat.

REPAIRING THE DAMAGE FAQ

■ WHAT IS PHILIP'S MOST IMPORTANT WEIGHT-LOSS RECOMMENDATION?

Eating real whole food is the number one change you can make to lose weight. Your sugar consumption will be cut close to zero, you'll eliminate processed foods like seed oils, and you'll avoid preservatives and other chemicals that can damage metabolic health. Changing your diet also makes every other metabolic change easier to follow.

■ IS IT TOO LATE TO START LIVING HEALTHY AFTER FORTY OR FIFTY?

Better metabolic health means better quality of life. There's no reason not to start, no matter how old you are. I've helped clients who are sixty, seventy, and even eighty years old improve their metabolic health and see good results from it.

The later you start, the more likely you are to already have some damage. That damage may or may not be reversible, but you can stop it from getting worse. The sooner you start, the better.

If you're seventy years old and miserable because of your metabolic health, fixing it now means you may reach your eighties or nineties and experience a better quality of life as you age. If that gives you twenty more years with your family instead of two more years, you'll get to witness—and impart your wisdom to—a whole extra generation.

IS IT POSSIBLE TO NOT ONLY RESET YOUR BODY BUT REVERSE DAMAGE CAUSED BY LIFELONG POOR EATING HABITS?

Some damage is reversible, some is not. You can't undo a heart attack you've already had, for example. But even if you have damage that is not reversible, improving your metabolic health can stop the issues from getting worse.

For example, there have been individual cases of people lessening coronary artery calcium scores, but we don't have good evidence of that happening on a large scale—yet. We have more evidence for slowing the natural progression of disease and decline.

For example, people with CAC typically see an increase of 10 to 20 percent every year. If you stop that increase or at least slow it down, you can expect better overall health compared to the otherwise natural decline and increased risks.

It is always better to improve your metabolic health. You can reverse any damage that's reversible, and your quality of life will improve even if some damage remains.

CAN IMPROVING METABOLIC HEALTH REVERSE TYPE 2 DIABETES?

Type 2 diabetes is the biggest, brightest red flag that it's time to change. Conventional belief is that once you have it, you'll never be healthy again. But type 2 diabetes is not a lifelong condition, and it can be reversed.

Follow the advice in this book diligently. The worse your metabolic health, the stricter you may need to be with these principles. But you can absolutely reverse this disease and free yourself from insulin dependence.

SOCIAL CONCERNS FAQ

▪ HOW DO I DISCUSS MY DIETARY CHANGES WITH PEOPLE?

You should eat in the way that allows you to best achieve your goals. Other people's opinions should have no bearing on this decision. However, your family and friends may express initial concern when they hear you're shifting to a radical new eating plan. They've probably heard all kinds of food industry talking points and may be genuinely alarmed for your well-being.

If you get some pushback from a spouse or other loved ones, explain that you're going to try this new eating plan as a means of improving your quality of life. Share some of the metabolic health markers you'll be monitoring as you progress. Explain that you'll be open with your results and will drop the plan if your health worsens. Then ask for their support as you investigate your options.

Results are the best argument for your choices. If you are improving your health and feeling and looking better, then who cares what anyone who doesn't support your eating choices thinks? Don't let people with terrible metabolic health tell you what's healthy for you.

▪ HOW CAN I MAINTAIN MY WAY OF EATING IN SOCIAL SITUATIONS?

Every society has food-centric social events. People gather and expect you to eat with them. If you don't, they might think something weird is going on, or you might perceive that others are judging you.

I get it. Other people exert a lot of pressure for you to eat the way they think you should. Especially at social events. What is a metabolically healthy way to approach these events?

Advance planning is your friend. Ask the event coordinator what they're going to serve. Don't worry, most people ask that question. Plan which foods you will and will not eat beforehand.

Don't show up starving. That's a sure way to binge on the wrong foods. Eat in advance of the social event so you're reasonably full. That way you can control exactly what you do and don't want to consume.

Minimize your alcohol consumption. Drink water or club soda instead. This will also help you detox from social drinking.

If people ask why you are eating so little or nothing, it's OK to just say you're not hungry without discussing your way of eating. You don't owe an explanation to anyone. You can even say you got hungry earlier and ate before you came. If the pressure is too intense, and if you really did eat before the event like I recommended, you can get away with eating just a small amount of unhealthy food.

Keep in mind that your enjoyment in life shouldn't be focused on food. Spending time with your friends and family should be what's important. Food at social events just makes sure everyone is content and won't need to leave to find something to eat. Let food serve as a vehicle for social engagement instead of taking center stage and replacing human interaction as the most important part of the celebration.

It's OK to have some food that is "off plan" from time to time in limited amounts. I do this myself on occasion. One unhealthy meal won't destroy your life. I tell my clients to first of all not view it as "cheating." No one sticks to a plan 100 percent. "Allowing yourself the indulgence" is a better way to phrase it.

The key is to get back to sticking with the plan the next day and to make the majority of your days healthy ones.

HOW CAN I HELP CONVINCE FAMILY AND FRIENDS TO CARE ABOUT THEIR METABOLIC HEALTH?

It's incredibly hard to make people care. It's also difficult to convince them they've been living inside a medical system that secretly keeps them sick to farm them for money.

Instead, set an example. Get metabolically healthy, look great, and live a more active life. Your family and friends will notice and become envious. They'll crave to learn your secret. When they ask, then you can explain. Even if they have a hard time believing at first, you'll have the results to prove your claims. It's hard to argue with a fit waistline and huge muscles.

DEALING WITH DOCTORS FAQ

HOW DO I CONFIDENTLY NAVIGATE NUTRITION INFORMATION THAT DEVIATES FROM THE MAINSTREAM NARRATIVE OF "WHAT IS HEALTHY?"

It's important to recognize there is no perfect nutritional answer that fits everyone. You need to find what works for you by tracking the right metrics, such as the metabolic health parameters.

That said, on a large-scale societal level, it's clear that mainstream nutritional advice is not working. Any change you can make in a healthy direction will help. But it will require you to test your results and see how you react to different approaches. Focus on results to measure how your diet plan is working.

If you keep hearing about a fad diet, it does not make that diet healthy. The most heavily promoted message is not necessarily true. Often, heavy promotion means it's *not* true. You'll have to do some sense-making to get through the noise and find where the signal is coming from.

Look for qualifications and red flags. If the diet has a basis in metabolic health, pay close attention. If it advocates less fat and salt while ignoring sugar, it's probably wrong.

It's ultimately up to individuals to find what works for them. You need to seek out knowledgeable people to work with and learn from. Now that you understand the basic principles of metabolic health, it will be easier to figure out who is telling you the truth.

HOW CAN I TALK TO MY DOCTOR ABOUT LOW-CARB, KETO, AND CARNIVORE DIETS?

A lot of people get nervous about talking to the doctor. They imagine they'll sound crazy rattling off facts they heard on the internet, or that medical professionals will roll their eyes at them for being proactive.

The truth is, it should be easy to talk to your physician or healthcare professional. You don't have to put up with any antagonistic relationship.

Your physician should be glad you're taking an interest in your health and working to live longer. Both of you should want to keep you alive for as long as possible with the best quality of life achievable.

Tell your physician you want to discuss your health improvement goals. Explain that you're working on a whole life overhaul because you want to maximize your quality of life. That prevents you from sounding like you're just temporarily alarmed from a news story you heard.

As you work with your physician to improve your health, focus on improvements in your overall health instead of being overly concerned with one measure. Prioritize risk reduction.

If you're worried about getting pushback from a physician who doesn't understand metabolic health, present information that supports your choices. If your doctor won't even consider this information, find a new physician.

HOW DO YOU GET A PHYSICIAN TO ORDER A CORONARY ARTERY CALCIUM SCAN WHEN YOU CHOOSE NOT TO TAKE STATINS, WHICH MY DOCTOR PRESCRIBED?

The most recent guidelines from the American Heart Association recommend CAC scores for people at low or medium risk of heart disease, particularly when their only real risk factor is elevated cholesterol level. If you struggle to get your doctor to agree to CAC scores, you can point to those guidelines.

A physician has no reason to resist ordering CAC scores. True, they are not covered by insurance for the most part, but they can usually be done for under two hundred dollars and only take about five minutes. They involve a low dose of radiation, and they don't require any contrast or an IV.

I think these tests are woefully underutilized. If your physician is averse to CAC scores or other metabolic health concerns, the only answer may be to find a new one.

OVADIA HEART HEALTH FAQ

HOW IS DR. OVADIA'S MEDICAL PRACTICE DIFFERENT FROM TYPICAL CONCIERGE TELEMEDICINE?

Ovadia Heart Health is a holistic, comprehensive, and metabolic-health-first telemedicine practice. Most physicians focus on one area of health and prescribing drugs to address symptoms. That means they clean up after problems rather than fixing them.

Those kinds of practices leave your health problem running silent with all your warning alarms turned off. That's how skinny people die from heart issues.

My background as a heart surgeon has given me a unique insight into heart disease. I founded my practice on the principle that heart disease—and most other diseases—stem from metabolic disorders. At Ovadia Heart Health, we listen to patients' metabolic health concerns when other doctors won't, because we understand.

So if you need a doctor who listens, hears you, and can help, feel free to reach out. Book your free fifteen-minute session with me, the author, at **ovadiahearthealth.com**. The only regret people have about improving their metabolic health is waiting to do so.

METABOLIC HEALTH FOR LIFE

A good friend of mine is a nurse anesthetist at the hospital where I worked before opening my metabolic health clinic. You recall I was an overweight heart surgeon. My friend, too, struggled with weight and health problems. When we split up and went to different hospitals, we kept in touch to provide much-needed encouragement and accountability.

Then I started learning about metabolic health. My journey took me years, and whenever I'd connect with my friend, he noticed results taking shape. He saw pictures on social media, noticeable weight loss, and read what I said about low-carb eating. When he saw the success I was having, he reached out and asked, "What are you doing?"

This was my very first attempt to teach someone else all that I'd learned. He was a sort of proto-client for my fumbling attempts to articulate my new knowledge and insights about metabolic health. He had an accelerated journey because I walked him through what I did and helped him avoid what hadn't worked.

My friend listened patiently and did everything I suggested. First, he cut down on carbs and sugars. Second, he cut out vegetable and seed oils. Third, he moved to real whole foods: nuts, veggies, meats. Fast forward in his process, and he was able to fit into his basic training uniform he'd worn at eighteen. Like me, he had more energy and could keep up with his hockey player son.

Watching him heal and grow, I knew for certain that my journey hadn't been a fluke. I'd discovered the truth about how our bodies work. And I'd built a replicable method for healing people afflicted with metabolic sickness.

Being in the medical system, my friend has come to a lot of the same conclusions I have. And he has many of the same burning questions. Why doesn't the medical system talk about and use this more? Why are donuts and cookies everywhere in the hospital? Why are we only treating the symptoms of metabolic health and not the actual problems? Why are doctors fed so many lies, and why are they still teaching those same lies to their patients?

I still shake my head at how blind most medical practitioners are to the truth. A hospital will celebrate Doctors Day every March 30 with high-sugar, high-carb food instead of healthy foods like steak, lobster, or fresh vegetables. It's almost as if they want their own staff to be sick.

The same is true of our culture at large. We celebrate food at holidays instead of celebrating our family. Food can be a wonderful addition to that family celebration, but we've started to worship the food itself. Some people live for their next sugar fix. They don't even realize what's being done to them by the food industry. And doctors are just as confused as their dying patients.

Working with my friend opened my eyes to a great need in the world. Our experience demonstrated that what I say resonates with other people, that people are looking for this information, and that even healthcare professionals don't know the truth. I realized how needed this information is.

That's why I wrote this book. And I'm so glad you read it. Because now you can get metabolically healthy, too.

YOUR NEXT STEPS

As a heart surgeon, as a medical professional, as a health coach, and as a human being, I have a duty to help people prevent themselves from needing my heart surgery services. That means I need to spread the truth: what you eat determines your health. And the best thing to eat is real whole food where the food itself is the ingredient.

As we went through in this book, we discussed a lot of "fad diets" out there that seem to have good information. But if you go to other sources, you'll find good science disputing those facts. Figuring out the best real whole food for *you* to eat is the number one thing most of my clients want help with. They aren't sure how to take that next step, or they need personalized troubleshooting along the way.

That gets to the question of working with a cheap health coach or a heart surgeon. I have a full-spectrum picture because I work on both ends of the problem, the beginning and the end. I can legally review your lab work. And I know what heart disease—the top killer in America—is, and I know how to find the signs of it years in advance.

Your health is worth the investment. I work a lot with business executives and entrepreneurs. They always ask how much value I can provide for my cost. I ask them, "How much money would you make if you had five more years of productivity? If you could be more productive and efficient while you're working? How much more would that be worth? What are five more years with your family, spouse, kids, and grandkids worth to you?"

The price of your food is a small portion of the cost. The long-term cost needs to be recognized as well. It might be a smart investment to hire someone like me to coach you through this process so you maximize your results in the shortest amount of time. That way, you can get back to living and make every second count. If you agree . . .

- Follow me on Twitter **@ifixhearts**
- Follow me on Instagram **@ovadia_heart_health**
- Sign up for my email newsletter at **ovadiahearthealth.com**
- Take the Metabolic Health Plan course at **ovadiahearthealth.com**

- Or skip all the above and book a free session with me at **ovadiahearthealth.com**. (For companies, I offer group coaching to employees. That keeps your staff healthy and more productive.)

Follow this information in this book, and if you'd like specific guidance for your personal situation from me, let's talk.

IF YOU FORGET EVERYTHING ELSE, REMEMBER THIS

You don't have to end up on my operating table. Bad metabolic health is preventable.

I recently performed open-heart surgery and found the patient's heart encased in a layer of visceral fat. There is normally some fat on the heart, but muscle should at least be visible. Healthy human hearts should not be encased in fat. This patient's heart looked like a lump of fat as opposed to a muscle. I know that if I opened this patient's abdomen, I would find visceral fat encasing other internal organs, too. And that's another sure sign of metabolic disease.

What brought this person here was entirely preventable. Twenty or thirty years ago, if someone had told this man the information in this book, his heart would look a lot different—and I wouldn't be staring at it and photographing it today.

Ten years ago, I looked at all the same hearts, saw all the same fat, and thought it a nuisance. Because that fat makes it hard to access the blood vessels of the heart. Almost all the hearts I operated on looked like that, so I figured it was normal. But now, having this information, I realize this was preventable. It's years and years of buildup that could have been intervened on. I see these hearts as tragic examples of people fed lies, patients who never had a chance because they didn't have the truth.

But you do have the truth. This is your call to action. Remember that your metabolic health is fixable. Seven of the ten top causes of death in the

United States are metabolic. Take an active role in your metabolic health, and you can largely reduce the risk of them all.

Please take care of yourself. Don't end up on my table. I want you to have decades of high energy with your family.

You have what you need to get metabolically healthy. Go save your own life.

ACKNOWLEDGMENTS

Getting to the point of writing a book is not a journey one makes alone. There have been many along the way who have helped and guided me, and it is not possible for me to list them all.

My mother, Rebecca, and my father, Herman, taught me the essential life lesson to always strive to improve the world around you and the lives of those that you interact with. My sister, Nicole, and brother, Seth, have always been available for support and encouragement.

I have been fortunate during my medical training and career to have many mentors and partners. Included in this group are Francis Rosato (deceased), Reuven Rabinovici, Andrew Boyarsky, Kenneth Warner, and Alexander Vasilakis.

My personal and professional journey toward realizing the importance of metabolic health has been influenced and assisted by Tro Kalajian, Brian Lenzkes, Shawn Baker, Dave Feldman, and Jeff Grindstaff. I would also like to thank Casey Means for her contributions to the sections on metabolically healthy veganism.

And, most recently, establishing and growing Ovadia Heart Health has only been possible with the assistance of Brian Keith, Chris Cornell, Richard White, Joshua Lisec, Jack Heald and Jack Murphy.

Last, but not least, is a thank-you to all the patients who have entrusted me with their lives. Interacting with every one of them has been educational and humbling.

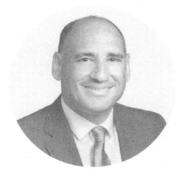

ABOUT THE AUTHOR

D r. **Philip Ovadia** is a board-certified cardiac surgeon and founder of Ovadia Heart Health. His mission is to optimize the public's metabolic health and help people stay off his operating table. As a heart surgeon who used to be morbidly obese, Dr. Ovadia has seen firsthand the failures of mainstream diets and medicine. He realized that what helped him lose over one hundred pounds was the same solution that could have prevented most of the thousands of open-heart surgeries he has performed—metabolic health.

In *Stay Off My Operating Table: A Heart Surgeon's Metabolic Health Guide to Lose Weight, Prevent Disease and Feel Your Best Every Day*, Dr. Ovadia shares the complete metabolic health system to prevent disease.

Dr. Ovadia grew up in New York and graduated from the accelerated Pre-Med/Med program at the Pennsylvania State University and Jefferson Medical College. This was followed by a residency in General Surgery at the University of Medicine and Dentistry at New Jersey and a Fellowship in Cardiothoracic Surgery at Tufts–New England Medical School.

Learn more about Dr. Ovadia at **ovadiahearthealth.com**.